Global Re-Visions

EDITED BY

Shampa Biswas, Bruce Magnusson, and Zahi Zalloua

T0355754

University of Washington Press

Seattle and London

IN ASSOCIATION WITH

Whitman College

Walla Walla, Washington

Global Re-Visions

This series aims to pursue the challenges that globalization poses, and the possibilities that it offers, in an interdisciplinary setting. Each volume seeks to promote a more nuanced understanding of timely issues while providing critical dialogue with prior scholarship and new ways of shaping how these issues are envisioned and framed. The series probes to what extent our vision of globalization both alters and is altered by the singularity and complexity of the topic at hand, compelling, in turn, perpetual re-visions.

Torture: Power, Democracy, and the Human Body
edited by Shampa Biswas and Zahi Zalloua

Contagion: Health, Fear, Sovereignty
edited by Bruce Magnusson and Zahi Zalloua

CONTAGION

HEALTH, FEAR, SOVEREIGNTY

EDITED BY

BRUCE MAGNUSSON

ZAHI ZALLOUA

University of Washington Press

PO Box 50096,

Seattle, WA 98145, USA

www.washington.edu/uwpress

Whitman College

345 Boyer Ave.

Walla Walla, WA 99362

www.whitman.edu

Library of Congress Cataloging-in-Publication Data

Global Studies Symposium on Contagion (2010 : Whitman College)

Contagion : health, fear, sovereignty / edited by Bruce Magnusson and Zahi Zalloua.

    p. cm. — (Global re-visions)

Papers presented at the Global Studies Symposium on Contagion held at Whitman College, Walla Walla, Washington, on Feb. 27, 2010.

Published in association with Whitman College, Walla Walla, Washington.

Includes bibliographical references and index.

ISBN 978-0-295-99174-0 (hardcover : alk. paper)

ISBN 978-0-295-99173-3 (paperback : alk. paper)

1. Bioterrorism—Congresses.   2. Bioterrorism—Health aspects—Congresses.

3. Disaster medicine—Congresses. 4. Terrorism—Prevention—Congresses.

I. Magnusson, Bruce A. II. Zalloua, Zahi Anbra, 1971– III. Title.

HV6433.3.G557 2010   363.325'3—dc23

2012002568

Printed and bound in the United States of America

Designed by Ashley Saleeba

Composed in New Baskerville and Franklin Gothic

The paper used in this publication is acid-free and meets the minimum requirements of American National Standard for Information Sciences—Permanence of Paper for Printed Library Materials, ANSI Z39.48–1984.∞

CONTENTS

ACKNOWLEDGMENTS

This volume emerged out of the Global Studies Symposium on Contagion held at Whitman College, Walla Walla, Washington, on February 27, 2010. Organized by the Global Studies Initiative, the symposium was developed to stimulate an interdisciplinary conversation on a topic of contemporary relevance. It appears to us that too many of our most important conversations happen within the relatively narrow confines of academic disciplines or specialist communities. Inspired by the liberal arts model of colleges like Whitman, we believe that it is both possible and valuable to generate discussions across different kinds of epistemic communities without sacrificing intellectual rigor. Our hope is that this volume, much like the symposium, will help generate a critical public debate on the role of contagion-thinking in global issues and will do so in a way that is both sophisticated and accessible to various reading publics. Andrew Lakoff, Priscilla Wald, and Alberto S. Galindo participated in the symposium and contributed revised versions of their presentations to this volume. We are also grateful to Stephen Morse and Jason Pribilsky for their substantial contributions to the symposium discussions and the development of our own thinking about contagion.

Our foremost gratitude goes to the many faculty, administrators, students, and staff who have helped make Whitman College the vibrant intellectual community in which projects such as these are possible. We would like to thank President George Bridges and Provost and Dean of Faculty Timothy V. Kaufman-Osborn for all their encouragement and support. Special thanks go to Shampa Biswas, Global Studies Director (2008–10), who spearheaded the vision for the symposium. We are also indebted to the other members of the Global Studies steering committee, Gaurav Majumdar (English), Jim Russo (Chemistry), and Elyse Semerd-jian (History), for their intellectual rigor in helping to conceptualize and implement this project. Susan Bennett, administrative assistant to the provost and dean of faculty, provided crucial logistical support all along the way. Nicole Simek read multiple versions of the introduction to this volume and provided insightful and crucial commentary and advice. Above all, none of this would have been possible without the enthusiasm and interest of the smart and dedicated students of Whitman College. Among these, we owe particular thanks to several whose contributions are reflected in many ways in this volume. Pre-med and Latin American Studies major DeeDee McCormick (2010), Biology major Nicole West (2010), and History major Seth Bergeson (2010) all participated in the symposium, and many of the chapters in this volume were enriched by their sharp commentary. Gender Studies major Spencer Janyk (2010), History major Omar Ihmoda (2011), and English major Gabriella Friedman (2013) provided invaluable research and editing support. We cannot emphasize enough how instrumental these and other students were in posing probing questions, challenging the contributors to sharpen their analyses, and in general elevating the quality of the symposium and the resulting volume through their active engagement. As teachers at Whitman College, we consider ourselves fortunate to be in the midst of such thoughtful and supportive colleagues and students. Finally, we would like to thank Pat Soden, Marilyn Trueblood, and Jacqueline Ettinger for all their encouragement and help with this volume.

We would like to express our gratitude for permission to reprint Paul B. Stares and Mona Yacoubian's "Rethinking the War on Terror: New Approaches to Conflict Prevention and Management in the Post-9/11

World," in *Leashing the Dogs of War: Conflict Management in a Divided World*, edited by Chester A. Crocker, Fen Osler Hampson, and Pamel Aall (Washington, D.C.: United States Institute of Peace Press, 2007), and Geoffrey Whitehall's "The Aesthetic Emergency of the Avian Flu Affect," in *Geopolitics of American Insecurity: Terror, Power, and Foreign Policy*, edited by François Debrix and Mark Lacy (New York: Routledge, 2009).

CONTAGION

INTRODUCTION

The Hydra of Contagion

Bruce Magnusson and Zahi Zalloua

Governments, scientists, politicians, doctors, law enforcement officials, journalists, gadflies, and others periodically alert us to potential devastation, potential catastrophe, an imminent moment of life and death resulting from a *successful* virus, whether the SARS virus of 2003 or HIV/AIDS for the last three decades, Communists in the 1950s, the hairtrigger possibility of nuclear war, a terrorist with the right weapon, irreversible invasions of documented and undocumented immigrants, an awakening sleeper cell in a bedroom community, or a cyber-terrorist capable of rendering helpless a multitrillion-dollar defense system. In 2009, we watched, organized, practiced, and inoculated as the country and the world were alerted to the potential catastrophe of a new H1N1 influenza virus. Global, national, state, and local institutions, businesses, communities, colleges, and prisons all organized themselves around the identification, surveillance, and control of that particular virus. More importantly, they developed contingency plans of enormous proportion for the potentially uncontrollable and unmanageable threat. We are warned; we organize; we practice; we adjust to the "new" circumstances. We do so out of fear of everything from historical memories of the 1918 influenza pandemic, which killed more than 50 million people worldwide, to the more contemporary reading of the September 11 attacks on the World Trade Center and the Pentagon as an infection of what is referred to as "radical Islam." A virus lies in wait, ready to breach the most elaborate hygienic, physical, intellectual, and moral defenses of sovereign states and sovereign individuals.

Over many decades, contagion has been a metaphor of choice for everything from global terrorism, suicide bombings, poverty, immigration, global financial crises, human rights, fast food, obesity, divorce, and homosexuality.[1] The unprecedented proliferation of contagion as a heuristic tool or interpretive category should give us pause, however. What happens to the concept of contagion when it exceeds its original epidemiological context and starts *contaminating* other discourses in the social sciences and humanities? Is this contamination to be celebrated as a positive effect of cross-fertilization, that is, for the cross-disciplinarity that it affords? Or do we need to scrutinize more carefully the ideological underpinnings of its dissemination in contemporary debates (keeping in mind who defines contagion and what or who gets defined as contagious)? Does an affirmative answer to the latter question render the former moot? We do not believe so. Contagion *as such* is to be neither celebrated nor condemned out of hand. Rather, we need to examine how the concept operates in a given system and fully explore its interpretive potential. To be sure, this is a daunting task. For this reason, a cross-disciplinary approach to contagion is not only useful but also necessary to understanding the complexity of contagion today. We have adopted the lenses of global studies in our examination of contagion. In doing so, however, we have taken care not to merely translate, apply, and/or transpose global insights onto the language of contagion. Rather, we propose to explore contagion not as an object of global interest but as a vexed trope for globalization itself, as a double-edged sword for thinking about global processes.

The Politics of Contagion/The Contagion of Politics

Understood as a particular kind of threat to the body, the body politic, the nation, global institutions, and the essential normative infrastructure of global life, contagion has served as a productive metaphor of globalization. But what are the consequences of the strategic enactment of institutional responses to biological contagions for thinking about security issues more generally? In chapter 1, "Rethinking the 'War on Terror': New Approaches to Conflict Prevention and Management in the Post-9/11 World," Paul B. Stares and Mona Yacoubian recommend "a counter-epidemic approach" to global terrorism.[2] Is contagion, then, contagious? Does it slip the containment of microbiology and enter other living realms of ideas, violence, fear, government, politics, and ethics? If so, how has it shaped our ways of thinking about, responding to, and reproducing global phenomena? More importantly, how does it shape our approach to organizing for the out-of-control? These questions are related to but travel beyond social contagion theory by asking how the inchoate fear of microbial disaster becomes a framework for larger questions about the nature and location of sovereignty and the related questions of contact and hygienic isolation, fear and invisibility, the hazards of sociability, the security of surveillance, and what a healthy security might mean.[3]

In *Emerging Viruses*, edited by Stephen S. Morse, Richard M. Krause sets the stage for thinking of contagion globally by beginning his foreword with a quote from Louis Pasteur: "Science knows no country because it is the light that illuminates the world." Krause both specifies and explodes Pasteur's dictum. "Like science," he says, "emerging viruses know no country. There are no barriers to prevent their migration across international boundaries or around the 24 time zones." As a response to the inevitability of future epidemics, which require surveillance, identification, and an enormous research effort, Krause concludes, "[T]o be successful, an effort of this complexity must be dominated by a *central concern* to curtail the nationwide, indeed worldwide, proliferation of an epidemic from an unexpected origin."[4] These comments, which introduce a 1993 book that by all accounts has changed the way in which scientists and policy makers perceive and respond to viral threats, are illuminating for our purposes in this volume. Viral contagion is always imminent, from sources human or exotically wild, unidentifiable and uncontainable within national boundaries until it is "too late," demanding enormous quantities of centrally, if not globally, managed funds and research as well as the institutionalization of global biopolitical strategies of surveillance, diagnosis, containment, eradication, and therapy.

Morse identifies three stages of emerging contagions: introduction, establishment, and dissemination.[5] He challenges biodiversity, an environmental ideal in need of protection from anthropogenic change. The capabilities and opportunities in the "zoonotic pool" for "potential emerging pathogens" are leveraged by the increasing opportunities globalization provides for human contact. "Think of these," Morse says, as "microbial explorers, discovering new niches—us—and exploring new territory."[6] Those niches in new territories are ever more rapidly accessible around the globe with the increasing density and speed of air travel, global trade, and the crossing of all boundaries, territorial and biological, especially through human contact with food animals.

How can societies protect themselves from such threats? Infrastructures of national vigilance are complicated by the failure of such viruses to respect national sovereignty. As Morse has suggested, "effective global surveillance is one [way of protecting], as are better diagnostics, political will to respond to these events, and research to help understand the ecology and pathogenesis of these 'new' infections and to help develop effective preventive or therapeutic measures."[7] Global surveillance mechanisms such as the Pro-MED warning system for viral outbreaks mirror early-warning systems developed to forestall outbreaks of famine and human conflict.[8] Over-containment and overreaction may actually succeed in isolating and preventing pandemic outcomes, while the failure of a virus to successfully disseminate in such a situation may deepen public complacency about the threat itself. Yet an infrastructure of surveillance, vigilance, and counter-epidemic action must itself be maintained in order to enable quick mobilization upon evidence of threat. To the extent that the mobilization of fear and anxiety is the necessary agar in which policy makers and community, national, and global health officials can produce the public support necessary for effective countermeasures, the public inoculation itself begins to resemble processes of contagion. In order to succeed, it disrupts familiar spatial and temporal patterns of everyday life in favor of a vast, rapidly networked, transnational assemblage of experts, things, ideas, and institutions. So, to Morse's binary of emergency versus complacency, an alternative optic would suggest that emergency and complacency are necessarily co-constituted. In fact, the emergency is always latent—like a virus, it is never fully destroyed. Perfect health is unattainable.

Stares and Yacoubian cite a speech by Richard Haass to the Council on Foreign Relations in which he draws the relevant analogy: "The challenge of terrorism is . . . akin to fighting a virus in that we can accomplish a great deal but not eradicate the problem." They suggest that an effective approach to addressing the challenge of "Islamist militancy," in contrast to the global war on terror, would be to understand the threat (for purposes of countering it) in terms of an epidemic. Conceding that, conceptually, many analysts have already applied the epidemiological metaphor to a variety of social phenomena (fashions, fads, rumors, civil violence, and revolutionary ideas), its application to Islamic militancy and terrorism becomes intuitive.

> Thus, references to terrorism being a "virus" or to al Qaeda "mutating"
> or "metastasizing" are common. Similarly, the image of madrassas and
> mosques being "incubators" of a "virulent ideology" is frequently invoked.
> Such metaphors have a visceral appeal in that they help convey a danger-
> ous and, moreover, darkly insidious threat. For some, the disease metaphor
> also sets—implicitly, at least—a more realistic goal for what can be practically
> achieved to eliminate this scourge.

The effortless move here from metaphorical and visceral danger to realism is remarkable for its simplicity and audacity, calling attention to the rigor of epidemiological research standards and methodologies and webs of direct and indirect causalities while recognizing that "success in controlling and rolling back an epidemic typically results from a carefully orchestrated, systematic, prioritized, multipronged effort to address each of its constituent elements." The epidemic model, which describes the connections between host, agent, environment, and vector, is transformed into "the epidemic model applied to terrorism," a move that eviscerates territorial sovereignty and the state as the unit of analysis in favor of, among other things, cells, organizations, mosques, social networks, and the Internet. The world is reimagined as a geography of bounded zones of containment, protection, and vulnerability. Sovereignty in its national form becomes an invisible and uncomfortable anomaly in the unstable play of ideationally defined threats, boundaries, minorities, and institutions.[9]

The effortlessness of the movement between epidemiological analysis, metaphors of contagion and their visualization, institutions of security, and the imagination and fears of global contact occupies a central place in this volume. How should we think about the ways in which seemingly objective, if unrealized, conditions of epidemiological contagion entail transformative ideological, institutional, cultural, and structural consequences? In their chapters, Andrew Lakoff and Geoffrey Whitehall give us two different but related perspectives on how to understand these phenomena.

The model of counterterrorist epidemiology that Stares and Yacoubian propose in chapter 1 resembles the global health security model of rationality that Lakoff distinguishes from an alternative model, which he calls "humanitarian biomedicine." The security model, he argues, focuses on preventing emerging, imminent, or unrealized outbreaks. The competing humanitarian biomedicine model, by contrast, aims to reduce suffering from diseases that already "afflict the poorer nations of the world, such as malaria, tuberculosis and HIV/AIDS." These two different rationalities result in very different institutional configurations and, ultimately, "ethical stances." In chapter 2, "Epidemic Intelligence: Toward a Genealogy of Global Health Security," Lakoff introduces a very different optic on the relationship between the virus, sovereignty, and a global capitalist hierarchy of distribution. At the same time, he draws our attention to the contingent qualities of the invisible metaphors and rationality of the viral security discourse. A focus on protection from the virus rather than on the human suffering it causes demonstrates how the power of imagined threats to a bounded and sovereign body can institutionally trump (in institutions of international cooperation as well) a focus on the human misery itself. Competing paradigms from different levels of analysis are a familiar problem in international politics. The difference in perspectives on the 2010 Haitian earthquake provides a similar example: Was the disaster a result of inadequate prevention in terms of engineering and infrastructure, or was the human toll a consequence of poverty and global inequality? How policy makers think about cause and effect will determine, in large part, the mobilization, organization, and deployment of policy, institutional, material, and cultural resources.

When the health security perimeter fences off much of the global South, demands for global equity in the fight against contagions confront security grids aimed at sealing off those parts of the world in which public health infrastructure is incapable of addressing an outbreak. Lakoff's intervention reorganizes this global imaginary in a way that counters the purity and isolation of the sovereign body with a prescription to transcend sovereignty's imagined vulnerabilities in the goal of healing the already universalized afflictions of "a common humanity." For, in a conflict between sovereignty and the virus, it is the global linkages across organizations, professions, and populations that can address the sovereign integrity of the virus. As the vectors of contagion assault not just imagined sovereignties, the virus becomes a new vector of capital and property that leaves vulnerable the structurally determined victims of the virus itself. In the example Lakoff cites, an Australian pharmaceutical company appropriated an Indonesian strain of the H5N1 virus for the production of a vaccine that would, because of its cost, be inaccessible to Indonesians. The question is, then, not only when cooperation becomes a security threat but who becomes secure and who becomes vulnerable in the cooperation game. Moreover, isolation and quarantine, in a context of leaky borders, reduce the sociability necessary for the implementation of cooperative counter-epidemiological policies.

In chapter 3, "The Aesthetic Emergency of the Avian Flu Affect," Geoffrey Whitehall takes a different approach to the competing models Lakoff presents. Whitehall interprets this shift from sovereignty organized around national life to sovereignty organized around human life not as a competing paradigm for understanding global health security but as a way of understanding the easy slippage among categories (within the realm of human security) due to the "antigenic shift" from national states of exception, in which national life, or the citizenry, is the object of protection, to international states of exception, in which humanity must be protected from its enemies. The territorial problem of identifying where a sovereignty of humanity might reside invites a redefinition of sovereignty that requires a new politics, visible through an aesthetic appreciation of fear itself as constitutive of the threat to humanity. This move requires replacing the concept of an infected nation that can be isolated through international sanctions, boycotts, or embargoes with the idea of infected life and the consequences for a security apparatus aimed not just at other states but at animals, viruses, and people who may threaten humanity itself (what happens, for example, when the pigs and chickens are all exterminated, but the virus lives on in human subjects?). *Citizenship* cannot generate the security apparatus of a state for protection against threats to *humanity*. Fear, for Whitehall, "*is* the affective governance of a preemptive state of emergency" and is not isolated from the affective governance that created those threats. For him, resistance to normalized relationships between law and life (a consequence of shifting sovereignty) as well as an appreciation of the aesthetic shift from citizen to humanity are necessary for the emergence of a politics that would disrupt the aesthetic inevitability of political paralysis and complacency in the face of a generalized and inchoate threat to humanity.

Epidemiology as Ideology: Figuring (Out) the Contagious Other

The paradigmatic epidemiological model of a healthy body fighting off a foreign entity proves to be ideologically pregnant in a number of unexpected ways. What constitutes a healthy organism, a truly sovereign (singular, collective, national and/or international) body? How does the self's investment in its well-being translate in terms of the ways in which it conceives of the external danger? What language is deployed to make sense of the self's exposure to this menacing other? Recourse to the familiar language of "friend" and "foe" is to some extent understandable. This antagonistic logic is so ingrained in public discourse that it has become a natural or naturalized response to a perceived threat—be it political or biological.

Despite their pursuit of objectivity, scientists and researchers are not immune to the infiltration of normative rhetoric in their discourse. The temptation to see microbes and viruses as extremely clever enemies, capable of infiltrating the most complex of immune systems—those of human beings, for example—is a very strong one. Some pursue this comparison further, asking whether microbes and viruses are merely the vehicles by which nature imposes its will on its subjects. In *Virus X: Tracking the New Killer Plagues*, for example, Frank Ryan describes viruses as nature's "knights," defenders that are "not primarily designed to attack humanity" but that respond aggressively to "human exploitation and invasion of every ecological sphere."[10] Isn't the current epidemic, or the promise of a future pandemic (experts keep reminding us that it is coming), evidence, then, of nature's war on humanity, so to speak? Simply stated, we are witnessing nature's punishment for our compromising of innumerable ecosystems and mismanaging the earth's precious resources. Here, interpreted holistically, nature's devastating behavior could still be construed, albeit counterintuitively, as nature's attempt to save us from our fallen selves.[11]

Conversely, the presence of infectious disease might point to an altogether different scenario. Perhaps we should interpret nature's revenge more accurately as nature's indifference or lack of concern for humanity. Isn't nature simply an amoral force that does not differentiate between its multiple creatures? Isn't one of Darwin's primary lessons that in the natural order of things *Homo sapiens* holds no privileged ontological position? Human beings, like members of any other species, fall subject to the whims or unpredictability of natural selection. To be sure, coping with this narcissistic wound has not been easy, and recourse to an anthropomorphic depiction of nature (posited in both cases as an agent, who either exacts revenge or expresses indifference) along with her army of devastating microbes and viruses can be seen as an attempt to make sense of man's precarious condition in a Darwinian, or post-human, world, one still dominated, incongruously, by a binary logic of friend or foe.

In chapter 4, "Bio Terror: Hybridity in the Biohorror Narrative, or What We Can Learn from Our Monsters," Priscilla Wald explores the manifestation of the dilemmas and challenges confronting today's researchers in popular fiction and film. For her, the subgenre of biohorror, also called "epidemiological horror," best embodies literature's ongoing engagement with the pressing issues of contagion in the context of globalization, which altered traditional ways of responding to contagious diseases. "Popular cultural forms," states Wald, not only "register the cultural anxieties and fascination that arise when scientific and technological innovations and geopolitical transformations introduce new ways of understanding the world" but also "characteristically dramatize, and in the process alter, new theories as they appear in specialist publications and conferences and reach the general public through the mainstream media." Such films and fiction do not, then, simply vulgarize new scientific theories and mimic the latest jargon about contagion but lend themselves to critical analysis, enabling the spectator, reader, or critic access to his or her culture's political unconscious.[12]

The subgenre of epidemiological horror exploits especially well the anxieties surrounding the interpretive difficulty of distinguishing the communicable disease from its unwitting victim: the contagious, monstrous other. Deciding who or what is the appropriate object of blame and fear—the infection or the infected—becomes a murky task when the ontological makeup of the host undergoes radical transformation. In Jonathan Maberry's 2009 novel *Patient Zero*, for example, the infected blend in so well in society that the discovery of their *hybrid* identity is deadly or, at the very least, traumatizing and terrorizing. Hermeneutic anxieties about the inability to differentiate the human from the monster abound in biohorror, but in the context of the post-9/11 war on terror, this phantasmatic threat of hybrids and monsters takes a new twist: the infected other becomes the terrorist par excellence.

Wald's analysis of hybridity, a concept that has received extensive treatment in theorizations of globalization, casts doubts on the view that globalization has assimilated difference and normalized the hybrid. In their 2000 landmark work *Empire*, Michael Hardt and Antonio Negri take such a position, for example, in arguing against a "politics of difference," claiming that in focusing on the "truth" of the other's difference, postmodernist and postcolonial theorists play into the hands of their enemy, who gladly celebrates difference: "This new enemy not only is resistant to the old weapons but actually thrives on them, and thus joins its would-be antagonists in applying them to the fullest. Long live difference! Down with essentialist binaries!"[13] By extension, the argument continues, hybridity—the once cherished strategy for combating identitarian boundaries and antagonisms—has become the new norm of globalization. As a result, the concept has lost its critical edge; hybridity can no longer serve as an effective means of resistance to the homogenizing force of globalization, since it is neutralized and absorbed by the very system it purports to contest. While it might be true that late capitalism has successfully co-opted certain forms of difference, biohorror narratives symptomatically translate persistent anxieties about difference, about the uncanny and contagious other. Such anxieties have only intensified since the onset of the war on terror.

The relation between biohorror and politics is not itself new. During the Cold War, Communism was often likened to a communicable disease menacing the world. Like healthy carriers who are highly deceptive in appearance, Communist spies were portrayed as bearers of ideological bacteria, infecting the minds of American civilians. While the current war on terror has not (yet?) produced the kind of hysteria witnessed during the McCarthy era, clear signs of heightened Islamophobia are appearing in the United States, particularly in the rhetoric of protesters and elected representatives. Representative Louie Gohmert of Texas, for example, spoke on the floor of Congress about an elaborate conspiracy theory wherein terrorist cells are breeding within U.S. borders so as to produce future American-citizen terrorists who would then enact their most nefarious plan—the destruction of the United States: "It appeared they would have young women who became pregnant [and] would get them into the United States to have a baby. They wouldn't even have to pay anything for the baby. And then they would return back where they could be raised and coddled as future terrorists. And then one day, 20, 30 years down the road, they can be sent in to help destroy our way of life."[14] It is easy to dismiss Representative Gohmert's fearmongering as limited to the right-wing fringe and thus not to be taken seriously. To do so, however, would be to minimize a growing climate of perpetual anxiety on the right, or, more precisely, among some members of the Tea Party, a climate under which *redefining* what it means to be "American" (in order to exclude those deemed improper infiltrators) is perceived as an urgent task. The rise of Islamophobia, seen most clearly in recent reactions to plans for an Islamic cultural center near Ground Zero in Manhattan (which, in turn, prompted Pastor Terry Jones to call for a Qur'an burning on the ninth anniversary of the 9/11 attacks), Arizona's SB1070 immigration bill, and the expressed wish by GOP leaders to "revisit" the Fourteenth Amendment, points to a certain fear of contagious otherness, an otherness perceived to be at odds with a fetishized image of national sovereignty, a "true"—that is, an undiluted, uncontaminated, and unchanging—American way of life.[15]

In the American imaginary, democracy and the American way of life are symbiotically interwoven; in public discourse, the latter could not exist without the full presence of the former. In addition to guaranteeing a way of life at home, American democracy, which is commonly evoked as synonymous with American exceptionalism, serves in this imaginary as a global antidote to the most corrupt and tyrannical governments in the world. To threaten the American way of life is thus to threaten the future of democracy itself, everywhere. Against the virus that is terrorism, American democracy has taken unexpected if not unprecedented actions to protect itself, including some that jeopardize democratic rule, turning the system against itself, so to speak. French philosopher Jacques Derrida draws on the biomedical notion of autoimmunity in order to account for the modern ambivalent state of democracy. In the process of autoimmunization, Derrida writes, "a living being, in a quasi-*suicidal* fashion, 'itself' works to destroy its own protection, to immunise itself *against* its 'own' immunity."[16] Autoimmunity in its original biological context signifies a disorder, a living organism's failure to recognize that it is attacking a very part of itself. Moving from the individual body to the political body, Derrida examines "this strange illogical logic"[17] of autoimmunity, as he calls it, in the U.S. response (its body politics) to the traumatic events of 9/11. In its desire to protect itself against the spreading disease of terrorism, the United States has turned against itself, against its own self-protection, against, that is, its immune system: laws aimed at safeguarding the legal rights of its subjects, especially during states of emergency.[18] In its fight against the virus of terrorism, American democracy, under the willful watch of the Department of Homeland Security, thus suppresses its own traditional mechanisms of auto-protection—and arguably compromises its own integrity—in favor of an alternative, hypervigilant mode of self-protection that must posit the United States in a state of perpetual war. In Machiavellian fashion, for instance, former deputy assistant attorney general John Yoo makes explicit the ideological shift in what constitutes military normalcy after 9/11: "The world after September 11, 2001 . . . is very different from the world of 1993. It is no longer clear that the United States must seek to reduce the amount of warfare, and it certainly is no longer clear that the constitutional system ought to be fixed so as to make it difficult to use force. It is no longer clear that the default state for American national security is peace."[19]

In the same spirit, we could say that it is also no longer clear that the default state for the U.S. legal system is due process. Take, for example, the egregious denial of habeas corpus rights for detainees, or, rather, "terrorist suspects," at Guantánamo Bay, Cuba.[20] To be sure, the U.S.

14

Constitution provides for the suspension of the writ of habeas corpus, but this option is reserved for truly exceptional situations: "The Privilege of the Writ of Habeas Corpus shall not be suspended, unless when in Cases of Rebellion or Invasion the public Safety may require it."[21] The putative necessity of an open-ended "war on terror" supersedes this fundamental legal protection, transforming an *exceptional* and *temporary* action into a far more *normal* and *permanent* condition. The USA Patriot Act, more generally, emblematizes this curtailing of individual civil liberties in the name of a greater good: American sovereignty.

15

Yet the unruly logic of autoimmunity exposes the delusional quality and self-destructive potential of thinking of sovereignty in such absolute terms. Derrida not only reveals the danger of a political body incapable of discerning its own cells (citizens) from pathogens (hybrids, contagious others) but unravels the "phantasmatico-theological"[22] character of sovereignty: "it is not some particular thing that is affected in autoimmunity but the self . . . that finds itself infected."[23] Moving back and forth between the individual body and the political body, Derrida, like Wald, foregrounds a kind of "hybrid sovereign," or what he calls a "*sovereign without sovereignty.*"[24] Making an analogy with a body's need for "immunodepressants" (functioning as a necessary "supplement" to the immune system) in order to counter its natural antibodies and render possible "the tolerance of certain organ transplants,"[25] Derrida stresses the self's lack of self-sufficiency and autonomy. But what follows from this heteronomous condition is neither despair nor nostalgia but an awareness of the relational quality of the self, an awareness of the self's exposure to otherness: "[A]utoimmunity is not an absolute ill or evil. It enables an exposure to the other, to *what* and to *who* comes—which means that it must remain incalculable. Without autoimmunity, with absolute immunity, nothing would ever happen or arrive; we would no longer wait, await, or expect, no longer expect one another, or expect any event."[26] Without autoimmunity, "the aesthetic/affective mode of governance" so eloquently described by Whitehall in chapter 3 would be even less vulnerable to challenges and contestations. Stated more positively, autoimmunity entails a different "form of rationality," to recall Lakoff's language—a rationality more hospitable to contagion, to the contagious other (the immigrant, for example)—whose effects on the self (the host, the democratic citizen) cannot be fully determined in advance.[27]

In chapter 5, "Contagion, Contamination, and Don DeLillo's Post–Cold War World-System: Steps toward a Haptical Theory of Culture," Christian Moraru investigates this ontological relation of being-with others in an age of globalization, focusing closely on the bodily dimension of this shared condition and its implications for an understanding of culture based on the problematic of the "haptical" (etymologically derived from the Greek *háptomai*, "to touch").[28] What happens to man's ontological condition of being-with others under the ever-expanding forces of globalization? Following Jean Baudrillard and other cultural theorists, Moraru takes the end of the Cold War as a historical marker for the proliferation of a different kind of touching, one whose logic of contamination functions to replicate the same across the world's irreducible field of difference, transforming, if not de-forming, the lived *world* into a homogenized *globe*. Far from announcing the collapse of ideological divisions, inaugurating a new age of democracy after the "end of history,"[29] Moraru first paints a rather bleak image of the processes of globalization. The virus of globalization—or, better yet, globalization as "a cultural-linguistic pandemic"—is totalizing in nature; rather than consisting of a genuine encounter in which contact results in alteration or transformation, globalization aggressively promotes a mode of touching that results in an asymmetrical economy of reproduction and one-sided communication.

Yet Moraru's analysis or diagnosis of globalization's sociocultural ills does not stop here. Turning to postmodern American novelist Don DeLillo, Moraru shows moments of interruption and disruption in the hegemonic globalization of Babel. For Moraru, DeLillo reminds us of language's irreducibility: how language always exceeds its ideological function, that is, its deployment in the service of the reduction of the world's linguistic multiplicity to the repetitive selfsameness of one global *logos*. Language remains a potential "agent of redemption," announcing the possibility of an alternate, and ultimately more dialogical, "cultural haptics." This alternative model is not sought in some uncontaminated space *outside* of globalization but *through* its very reproductive logic. Looking at DeLillo's fiction as a case study for postmodern haptics, Moraru underscores the author's aesthetic commitment to a more personalized form of linguistic repetition in which difference is reintroduced through intertextuality (the world as a body of recyclable bodies of texts), a creative rewriting, or, in the words of Klara, one of the artist figures from his 1997 novel *Underworld*, a "painting over" of conventional cultural-political patterns and codes. What emerges from DeLillo's novels are viral narratives that open up a space for rethinking cultural production, reproduction, and circulation of "new" ideas, for imagining a pluralistic and dynamic world (as opposed to a one-dimensional "global haptics") in which bodies touch, interact, and communicate with one another while preserving their singular identities.

Pursuing further the problematic of contagion as an interpretive trope, Alberto S. Galindo looks at the precariousness of ideological stances in post-9/11 fiction. In chapter 6, "Contagion of Intellectual Traditions in Post-9/11 Novels," Galindo assesses literature's responses to the tragedy of 9/11, focusing primarily on Claire Messud's *The Emperor's Children* (2006) and Zoë Heller's *The Believers* (2009). Taking as a point of departure Judith Butler's sobering warning about the rise of anti-intellectualism in the aftermath of 9/11—along with its correlative call for a return to the simple binary logic of good and evil—Galindo explores how these two novels stage their ambivalence toward the bourgeois notion of liberalism as an antidote to the spread of fear and intolerance of others (that is, Islamic others). Both novels effectively complicate the alleged moral and political superiority of the liberal position as embodied by its respective characters by either exposing their ideological complicity with the system they deride or by pointing out their blind spots: progressive ideas often take a backseat to the greater ideal of American prosperity in *The Emperor's Children*, for instance.

Writing against the grain—against the end of irony—the authors of *The Emperor's Children* and *The Believers* contaminate a dominant interpretive horizon characterized by a type of "seriousness" all too prevalent in a post-9/11 aesthetico-political sensibility. What is subjected to irony in these texts is not so much an ideological stance (although liberalism is a constant target) but the belief that ideology of any kind can function as an adequate mode of immunization, not only as a protection from outside threats but also as a strategy of self-containment that reinforces identitarian logic (immunizing oneself against self-doubt—yet another instance of the Derridean illogical logic of autoimmunity). In this respect, we can say that ideological critique itself is contaminated, subject to the play of irony: characters are rarely ideologically whole but

rather divided, holding contradictory positions, unharmoniously strad-
dling the private and the public, the personal and the collective.

Outline of the Volume

Designating someone or something as "contagious" involves ethico-
political judgments; contagion is rarely a value-neutral matter. In chapter 1, Paul B. Stares and Mona Yacoubian articulate their case for the
benefits of appropriating the language of epidemiology and its disease
metaphor in combating Islamist militancy. Treating terrorism as a disease that is, ideally, to be eradicated or at least, more practically, contained, Stares and Yacoubian shift attention away from the terrorist *as*
such to the environment and space in which anti-Western sentiment is
initially generated. From their perspective, madrassas and mosques function as "incubators" of a virulent anti-American ideology. Their solution
is arguably more modest and pragmatic than an abstract "global war on
terror": they advocate instead more attention to the economic and political conditions of the many disenfranchised Muslims in the Middle East
and across the world—those who are most vulnerable to the virus of
Islamist militancy. Improving general socioeconomic conditions as well
as encouraging political transparency, conflict management, and greater
respect for the rule of law will help immunize and protect further those
most prone to the disease in the first place.

In chapters 2 and 3, Andrew Lakoff and Geoffrey Whitehall critically
scrutinize the global health campaign, examining the ideological effects
of a more aggressive or preemptive attitude toward the threat of epidemics and pandemics. In a climate overdetermined by the anxieties
produced by the September 11 attacks, the United States' active promo-
tion of global health security has led to the emergence of "epidemic
intelligence" along with its own peculiar form of rationality, reconfigur-
ing how we think of infectious diseases. The primacy of global disease
surveillance over resource investment in places where actual suffering
is occurring reflects an ideological agenda, a hegemonic gesture toward
restructuring health matters around geopolitical needs. For Whitehall,
the success of this new global doctrine lies in its ability to manipulate and
govern people at the aesthetic-affective level, transforming us into subjects of fear. The authoritative story told by Western governments and

the mainstream media of an inevitable future catastrophe conditions us to expect the worst, making us more open to the implementation of new strategies of governance and surveillance.

What is at stake in these debates is the common good, designated as "*human* life," *universally* threatened. But whose common good is actually being defended—that of those who suffer abject living conditions, or that of would-be sufferers in wealthy nations? Is global health security an a priori good? Is a return to the nation and its interests (what proponents of *American* globalization dub "viral sovereignty") to be interpreted as detrimental to the health of globalization? Or is the "common humanity" championed by the more traditional model of humanitarian biomedicine to be preferred? Lakoff and Whitehall ultimately leave it to the reader to decide. What they make clear, however, is that the rhetoric of globalization—though appealing in its purported desire to overcome the narrow concerns of national self-interest in order to deal more effectively with emerging diseases—often hides and represses economic and political factors that harm a large of portion of humanity, denying them access to the current resources and benefits of globalization. Geopolitics thus not only informs but often conditions responses to real or imagined health crises. Whose healthy body is secured and whose body is left exposed are decisions rarely made in an ideological vacuum.

The authors of chapters 4, 5, and 6, Priscilla Wald, Christian Moraru, and Alberto S. Galindo, turn to films and novels as cultural works that not only illustrate but also enact the perplexities of contagion in a global context. For Wald, the popular subgenre of biohorror both thematizes and translates cultural anxieties about the unknown in a time of terror. This protean subgenre *adopts* the new vocabulary of epidemiology (the matter of new narratives and scenarios) but also *adapts* it, providing a dramatized account of the epidemiological scene that despite (or because of) its distortion allows us to grapple more productively with the many paradoxes produced by an encounter with the contagious other—figured as a monster, hybrid, and/or terrorist. Moraru explores the relation of contagion to globalization by revisiting the terms of the debate. How we relate to one another—as non-sovereign bodies in the world, as being-with others—under globalization has everything to do with the way we imagine and conceptualize globalization itself. With Don DeLillo's postmodern fiction, Moraru argues, a linguistic resistance to

globalization's economy of the Same takes place, enabling a resignifica-
tion of the lived world. Repetition with a critical difference also informs
Galindo's study of post-9/11 fiction. Considering a recently reinvigo-
rated Manichean logic of good and evil and an alleged return to serious
discourse, Galindo examines the ways in which contagion functions as
a trope for the reading process, when ideology critique itself becomes
contaminated by ironic play.

Irony's infectious potential serves as a timely reminder of contagion's
own resistance to conceptual containment and hermeneutic mastery.
Indeed, we could say that the globalization of contagion always risks
becoming a contagion of globalization: a continual proliferation of
recontextualizations and shifts in interpretive frameworks. This volume
considers such a risk not only an unavoidable consequence but also an
opportunity for reenvisioning globalizing processes.

NOTES

1   See, among others, Mia Bloom, *Dying to Kill: The Allure of Suicide Terror*
     (New York: Columbia University Press, 2005); and Andrew Robert
     Aisenberg, *Contagion: Disease, Government, and the "Social Question" in
     Nineteenth-Century France* (Stanford, Calif.: Stanford University Press,
     1999). With regard to immigration, the discourse of contagion was
     generated by the fear of disease itself and was eventually applied more
     metaphorically to cultural and national values. Archived editions of the
     New York Times from the mid-nineteenth century are illustrative. See also
     Nayan Shah's *Contagious Divides: Epidemics and Race in San Francisco's
     Chinatown* (Berkeley: University of California Press, 2001). For theories
     of financial contagion, see, among others, Franklin Allen and Douglas
     Gale, "Financial Contagion," *Journal of Political Economy* 108, no. 1 (2000);
     and Riordan Roett and Russell Crandall, "The Global Economic Crisis,
     Contagion, and Institutions: New Realities in Latin America and Asia,"
     International Political Science Review 20, no. 3 (1999). Jason Kirby quotes
     Angel Giuria, the secretary-general of the Organisation for Economic
     Cooperation and Development, who said in reference to European
     financial woes, "Contagion has already happened. This is like Ebola"
     (Jason Kirby, "Europe Gets Greeced," *MacLean's*, May 17 [2010], http://
     www2.macleans.ca/2010/05/07/europe-gets-greeced/). The media
     jumped on a 2009 study that suggested that divorce is contagious. See Rose
     McDermott, James H. Fowler, and Nicholas A. Christakis, "Breaking Up Is

Hard to Do, Unless Everyone Else Is Doing it Too: Social Network Effects on Divorce in a Longitudinal Sample Followed for 32 Years," October 18, 2009, SSRN, http://ssrn.com/abstract=1490708. Happiness, loneliness, obesity, and suicide have been similarly explained by social contagion theory. For a perspective on social contagion theory, see Paul Marsden, "Memetics and Social Contagion: Two Sides of the Same Coin?" *Journal of Memetics — Evolutionary Models of Information Transmission* 2, no. 2 (1998): 171–185. See Alison L. Hill et al., "Infectious Disease Modeling of Social Contagion in Networks," *PLoS Computational Biology* 6, no. 11 (2010): **21** 1–15. Nancy J. Knauer discusses a theory of homosexual contagion prevalent among anti-gay groups in "Homosexuality as Contagion: From the Well of Loneliness to the Boy Scouts," *Hofstra Law Review* 29, no. 2 (2000): 401.

2   Stares and Yacoubian's report was originally delivered for the United States Institute of Peace and is reprinted as chapter 1 of this volume.

3   While this is not a review of social contagion theory, its connection to network theory (and networks as the infrastructure of contagion) is instructive. See the online exchange between Eugene Thacker, "On the Horror of Living Networks," and Tony D. Sampson, "Contagion Theory Beyond the Microbe (and perhaps beyond networks too)," http://www. networkpolitics.org/request-for-comments/dr-thackers-position-paper. As Sampson suggests, networks, science, and media businesses are using what they learn from viruses for marketing and fad-creation purposes. See also Thacker's "Cryptobiologies," in Organicities, online node, *Artnodes*, no. 6, UOC, http://www.uoc.edu/ortnodes/6/dt/eng/thacker.pdf. (ISSN 1695–5951)

4   Richard M. Krause, foreword to *Emerging Viruses*, ed. Stephen S. Morse (New York: Oxford University Press, 1993), vii-xi.

5   Stephen S. Morse, "The Globalization of Infectious Diseases," talk delivered at the Whitman College Symposium on Contagion, February 27, 2009.

6   Ibid.

7   Ibid.

8   For an overview of early-warning mechanisms, institutions, and scholarship, see Herbert Wulf and Tobias Debiel, "Conflict Early Warning and Response Mechanisms: Tools for Enhancing the Effectiveness of Regional Organisations? A Comparative Study of the AU, ECOWAS, IGAD, ASEAN/ ARF and PIF," Working Paper no. 49, Crisis States Research Centre, London School of Economics Development Studies Institute, May 2009.

9   For another view, see Hendrik Spruyt, *The Sovereign State and Its Competitors* (Princeton, N.J.: Princeton University Press, 1994), for a discussion of

institutional isomorphism as a response to external and internal political and economic contingencies following a crisis of unit capacity. This analysis examines the institutional triumph of the sovereign state as the relatively uncontested unit of international politics. In this sense, then, institutional contagion is an adaptive response rather than a threat.

10   Frank Ryan, *Virus X: Tracking the New Killer Plagues — Out of the Present and into the Future* (Boston: Little, Brown, 1997), 320.

11   For Joshua Lederberg, the diseases affecting human life need to be understood as "'Nature's revenge,' for our intrusion into forest, irrigation projects, and climate change" ("Infectious Disease—A Threat to Global Health and Security," *JAMA* 276, no. 5 [August 7, 1996]: 417; see Priscilla Wald, *Contagious: Cultures, Carriers, and the Outbreak Narrative* [Durham, N.C.: Duke University Press, 2008], 39–42). Though the quotation marks around "Nature's revenge" alert the reader to an unconventional use of the expression, this line of thought ironically parallels Jerry Falwell's incendiary claim that AIDS is the product of divine engineering aimed at punishing both homosexuals and those who fail to condemn them: "AIDS is the wrath of a just God against homosexuals. . . . AIDS is not just God's punishment for homosexuals; it is God's punishment for the society that tolerates homosexuals." Quoted in Bill Press, "Press: The Sad Legacy of Jerry Falwell," *Millford Daily News*, May 18, 2007. In both cases, human suffering is explained teleologically: there is a purpose behind the suffering, an agent (Nature or God) behind the act (the spreading of the virus).

12   On fiction's role in helping to make this political unconscious more visible, see Ruth Mayer, "Virus Discourse: The Rhetoric of Threat and Terrorism in the Biothriller," *Cultural Critique* 66 (2007): 1–20.

13   Michael Hardt and Antonio Negri, *Empire* (Cambridge, Mass.: Harvard University Press, 2000), 138.

14   *Anderson Cooper 360*. CNN transcripts, http://transcripts.cnn.com/ TRANSCRIPTS/1008/12/acd.02.html.

15   The slogan "We want our America back," heard at summer 2009 anti-health care reform debates, is also emblematic of this nostalgia for a mystified past, which, in turn, translates into a deep suspicion that President Barack Obama is not one of "us"—he is a Nazi, a socialist, a Muslim, a Kenyan, an anti-colonial, and so on.

16   Giovanna Borradori, *Philosophy in a Time of Terror: Dialogues with Jürgen Habermas and Jacques Derrida* (Chicago: University of Chicago Press, 2004), 94.

17   Jacques Derrida, *Rogues: Two Essays on Reason*, trans. Pascale-Anne Brault and Michael Naas (Stanford, Calif.: Stanford University Press, 2005), 123.

18 For an alternative and more positive account of biopolitical immunity, see Roberto Esposito, *Bios: Biopolitics and Philosophy*, trans. Timothy Campbell (Minneapolis: University of Minnesota Press, 2008). For an insightful discussion of the similarities and differences between Derrida and Esposito, see Timothy Campbell, "Bios, Immunity, Life: The Thought of Roberto Esposito," *Diacritics* 36, no. 2 (2006): 6–11.

19 John Yoo, "War, Responsibility, and the Age of Terrorism," *Stanford Law Review* 57, no. 3 (2004): 816.

20 After the 2008 U.S. Supreme Court ruling on the *Boumediene v. Bush* case, **23** against the Bush administration and in favor of adequate due process for the detainees at Guantánamo Bay, the Bush administration started to send its "terrorist suspects" to facilities at Bagram Airfield in Afghanistan. The Obama administration, though it had expressed criticism of the Bush model, continues to implement this legally and morally dubious policy.

21 U.S. Const., art. I, § 9, cl. 2.

22 Jacques Derrida, "Peine de mort et souveraineté," *Divinatio* 15 (2000): 18.

23 Derrida, *Rogues*, 109.

24 Borradori, *Philosophy in a Time of Terror*, 191n14. Putting it in slightly different terms, Derrida writes: "What must be thought here . . . is this inconceivable and unknowable thing, a freedom that would no longer be the power of a subject, a freedom without autonomy, a heteronomy without servitude" (*Rogues*, 152).

25 Jacques Derrida, "Faith and Knowledge," in *Acts of Religion: Jacques Derrida*, ed. Gil Anidjar (New York: Routledge, 2002), 80n27.

26 Derrida, *Rogues*, 152.

27 In opposition to a rhetoric of hospitality, such as the one favored by France's right-wing politician Jean-Marie Le Pen, a rhetoric that only gestures to an openness to the other by privileging the latter's amenability to assimilation—"Le Pen's organicist axiom . . . only lets in what is homogeneous or homogenizable, what is assimilable or at the very most what is heterogeneous but presumed 'favorable': the appropriable immigrant, the proper immigrant"—Derrida embraces an infectious (understanding of) difference, a difference capable of changing France's ontological being by contaminating its mystified organic whole (Jacques Derrida, *Negotiations*, ed. and trans. Elizabeth Rottenberg [Stanford, Calif.: Stanford University Press, 2001], 102). Derrida (re)turns here to the radicality of the ethical biblical injunction "Love thy neighbor." What is demanded in this formulation is a love not only of the one who resembles me (the other as alter ego) but of the neighbor as stranger (the other as radical alterity). Contamination as an unsettling of the self's narcissistic complacency is constitutive of the ethical exposure to the other. Michael

Hardt and Antonio Negri transform the ethical Derridean model of love as a contamination of the self—that is, as an unsettling of its narcissistic complacency—into a full-blown political project. For Hardt and Negri, love is a contagious expression of profound generosity—"we need a more generous and more unrestrained conception of love." Michael Hardt and Antonio Negri, *Multitude: War and Democracy in the Age of Empire* (New York: Penguin, 2004), 351. Love represents a shift from the concern with the increase of the *self*'s power to act to a concern with *our* power to construct a new democracy: "Love does not end there [in the love for a particular other—spouse, mother, etc.]"; rather, "love serves as the basis for *our* political projects *in common* and the construction of a new society. Without this love, *we* are nothing" (ibid., 352; emphasis added).

28 See Jacques Derrida, *On Touching—Jean-Luc Nancy* (Stanford, Calif.: Stanford University Press, 2005).

29 See Francis Fukuyama, *The End of History and the Last Man* (London: Penguin Books, 1992).

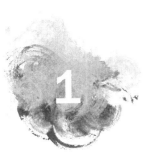

RETHINKING THE WAR ON TERROR

New Approaches to Conflict Prevention
and Management in the Post-9/11 World

Paul B. Stares and Mona Yacoubian

The new strategic challenge facing the United States in the wake of September 11 is often compared with the great "generational" struggles of the twentieth century against Fascism and Communism. While the contest likely will be as prolonged and require a comparable mobilization of national and international resources if the United States is to prevail, the comparison should not be pushed too far. The struggle in which we now find ourselves is like neither World War II nor the Cold War, with their clearly defined combatants, "front lines," and rules of engagement. The perpetrators of the September 11 attacks represent a transnational, highly dynamic, increasingly decentralized, religiously inspired movement propelled for the most part by a diverse collection of nonstate actors. They operate in some instances openly but more often clandestinely using unorthodox tactics and weapons. The challenge posed by what we define as "Islamist militancy" is fundamentally different, therefore, from traditional "state-centric" threats to international peace and security.

As such, Islamist militancy has more in common with other so-called new security challenges that transcend national borders and are driven by nonstate actors and processes. This does not mean that the traditional toolbox of national security responses is now irrelevant or renders obsolete the standard menu of conflict prevention and management techniques—on the contrary. But these techniques must be adapted and complemented with new approaches that acknowledge unconventional attributes of these new security challenges. In the case of Islamist militancy, the nature of the evolving challenge is still poorly understood. Thus, before describing an alternative, and what we believe to be a more effective strategy for responding to Islamist militancy than the approach currently favored in the global war on terror, this chapter lays out a different way of thinking about the new strategic challenge confronting the United States.

The New Strategic Challenge

Despite a plethora of studies and policy prescriptions since the September 11 attacks, we are still trying to grasp the nature of the new strategic challenge we face and how best to counter it. There is no better indication of this than the complete lack of consensus or common lexicon about what to call the threat. Is it "global terrorism," "Islamic terrorism," "al Qaeda and its affiliates," "Sunni jihadists," "Islamist radicals," or "terrorist extremism"? This is not just a semantics issue; words and names have vital operational import. Without clarity on who, precisely, is our adversary, we are unlikely to ever develop a clear and comprehensive understanding of its objectives, strategy, and operational character. And without such a common understanding, it will be difficult, if not impossible, to conceive of an effective and sustainable response. Yet it is our assessment that there is neither a broadly accepted understanding of the challenge we face nor a comprehensive long-term strategy for countering it.

Our preference is to classify this broader challenge as "Islamist militancy." Like the 9/11 Commission, we feel it important to use the modifier "Islamist," a politico-religious movement within the Muslim world, rather than "Islamic," the culture and religion of Islam.[1] Unlike the 9/11 Commission, however, we prefer the simpler, less loaded term "militancy" to "terrorism." Using the term "militants" to refer to those who either employ or espouse violent means in pursuit of political ends not

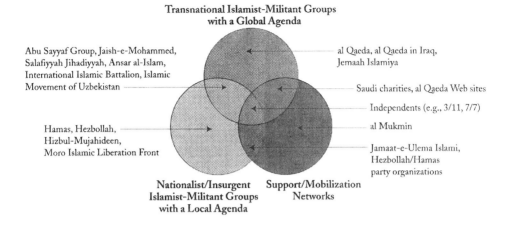

Transnational Islamist-Militant Groups
with a Global Agenda

Abu Sayyaf Group, Jaish-e-Mohammed,
Salafiyyah Jihadiyyah, Ansar al-Islam,
International Islamic Battalion, Islamic
Movement of Uzbekistan

al Qaeda, al Qaeda in Iraq,
Jemaah Islamiya

Saudi charities, al Qaeda Web sites

Independents (e.g., 3/11, 7/7)

Hamas, Hezbollah,
Hizbul-Mujahideen,
Moro Islamic Liberation Front

al Mukmin

Jamaat-e-Ulema Islami,
Hezbollah/Hamas
party organizations

Nationalist/Insurgent
Islamist-Militant Groups
with a Local Agenda

Support/Mobilization
Networks

1.1 Islamist Militancy, c. 2006

only avoids the notoriously slippery definitional problems associated with terrorism but also serves to underscore the multidimensional and broad-based nature of the challenge, involving more actors than just those who actually carry out terrorist attacks.[2] Indeed, Islamist militancy has three main constituent groups whose memberships are constantly evolving and overlap in significant ways.

There are, first, the transnational jihadist groups that have a global agenda (principally al Qaeda and its affiliates); second, the nationalist insurgent groups that have essentially a local agenda (e.g., Hamas, Hezbollah, and some of the Kashmiri groups); and, third, the miscellaneous organizations and networks that directly and indirectly support these militant groups. Distinctions among these groups are difficult to discern. Indeed, more and more new organizations and groups are emerging that share common traits and have overlapping agendas. Figure 1.1 provides a general snapshot of the principal actors in 2006. The diagram is not meant to be exhaustive and is merely illustrative of the phenomenon and its key constituent elements.

Islamist militancy does not represent a conventional national security threat—that much is clear and generally understood. Neither does it represent a conventional terrorist threat, which typically has a distinctive—often singular—identity with reasonably clear political goals, organizational structure, and area of operations. Conventional counter-terrorist responses, with their emphasis on apprehending an organization's leaders and rolling up networks or cells of activists and supporters through improved intelligence gathering and sharing, are therefore usually effective. Although such methods remain just as necessary to any campaign against Islamist militancy, it is also becoming clear that they will not be sufficient. The growing trend, exhibited in attacks such as those in Madrid (March 2004) and London (July 2005), for example, toward the emergence of localized, self-organizing militant groups acting largely independently of higher operational direction underscores the limits of conventional counterterrorism responses.

Not surprisingly, an increasing number of experts now advocate drawing on the strategies and tactics of unconventional, or "irregular," warfare to meet the challenge.[3] The threat is portrayed as a global insurgency that requires a commensurate global counterinsurgency (COIN) campaign. There is some logic to this view, as elements of the challenge reflect characteristics of a classic insurgency. Certainly, al Qaeda's stated goals of expelling "Jews and crusaders" from the Muslim world and cleansing it of apostate regimes—all with the objective of reestablishing a purified caliphate—can be viewed as an insurgency of sorts. The recognition that success ultimately hinges on winning "hearts and minds" in the Muslim world is also a critically important attribute of a counterinsurgency response.

Yet just as classic counterterrorism measures have their limits, so a strictly counterinsurgency approach has its shortcomings and even liabilities. Describing the phenomenon as a global insurgency dangerously exaggerates the threat by assuming a degree of organization and unity among its various actors that currently does not exist. The COIN approach also risks conflating many kinds of Islamist struggles and perversely even serving to legitimize them. Unless suitably adapted, the standard COIN framework with its simplistic distinctions between "enemies," "friends," and "uncommitted" could make matters worse, especially if military or "kinetic" responses come to dominate.

With these concerns in mind, we propose an alternative strategy for countering Islamist militancy that views the challenge as one would a global public health threat or epidemic. The conceptual leap required by this approach is not as far as it first appears. Social scientists increasingly have looked to epidemiology in order to understand a variety of social contagions, and, here, Islamist militancy is no different. Specifically, our approach draws on the scientific principles and practices of epidemiology as well as insights from a growing body of research on "social contagion phenomena" such as fashions, fads, rumors, civil violence, and revolutionary ideas.[4] Moreover, many commentators and even U.S. officials have employed disease metaphors to describe the challenge of Islamist militancy.[5] Thus, references to terrorism being a "virus" or to al Qaeda "mutating" or "metastasizing" are common. Similarly, the image of madrassas and mosques being "incubators" of a "virulent ideology" is frequently invoked. Such metaphors have a visceral appeal in that they help convey a dangerous and, moreover, darkly insidious threat. For some, the disease metaphor also sets—implicitly, at least—a more realistic goal for what can be practically achieved in attempting to eliminate this scourge. Just as very few diseases have been completely eradicated, so the likelihood that terrorism or political violence will be rendered extinct is remote. The best that can be hoped for is that it will become a manageable, low-probability, albeit sometimes deadly, nuisance much like many other social ills.

Beyond its metaphorical appeal, an epidemiological and public health approach offers more practical attractions, three of which stand out.

> » First, epidemiologists observe rigorous standards of inquiry and analysis in order to understand the derivation, dynamics, and propagation of a specific disease. In particular, they seek clarity on the origins and geographical and social contours of an outbreak: where the disease is concentrated, how it is transmitted, who is most at risk or "susceptible" to infection, and why some portions of society may be less susceptible or, for all intents and purposes, immune. Applying the same methodological approach to mapping and understanding Islamist militancy can yield immediately useful guidance on where and how to counter it.
>
> » Second, epidemiologists recognize that diseases neither arise nor spread in a vacuum. They emerge and evolve as a result of a complex dynamic interactive process between people, pathogens, and the environment in which they live. Indeed, the epidemiological concept of "cause" is rarely if ever singular or linear but is more akin to a "web" of direct and indirect factors that play a lesser or greater role in differing circumstances. To make sense

of this complexity, epidemiologists typically employ a standard analytical device that deconstructs the key constituent elements of a disease. This model helps not only in understanding the phenomenon in its entirety but also in anticipating how it might evolve in the future. The same systemic conception of disease can be adapted to understand the constituent elements of Islamist militancy and their evolution.

» Third, just as epidemiologists view disease as a complex, multifaceted phenomenon, so public health officials have come to recognize that success in controlling and rolling back an epidemic typically results from a carefully orchestrated, systematic, prioritized, multipronged effort to address each of its constituent elements. At the same time, however, it is also recognized that significant progress or major advances can sometimes be precipitated by relatively minor interventions—or "tipping points."[6] Again, there are lessons and insights to be learned here for orchestrating a global counterterrorism campaign.

Before turning to what such a campaign to defeat Islamist militancy might look like were it to follow a public health or counter-epidemic approach, it is necessary to understand how epidemiologists typically try to understand disease and how this can help us understand the challenge we face.

The Epidemic Model

As indicated, epidemiologists employ a standard approach, or model, to study epidemics that deconstructs an outbreak into four key components, recognizing that they are all dynamically interconnected, as shown in figure 1.2.[7]

In simple terms, the agent is the pathogen (e.g., a virus or bacterium) that causes disease. The host is the person infected with the disease (the "infective"), while the environment is composed of a variety of external factors that affect both agent and host. At the center of the triad are the vectors, the key pathways, or conduits, that help propagate the disease.

Islamist militancy is clearly not a disease in a comparably clinical fashion. Whereas those who fall victim to disease are typically passive and unwitting receptors of the pathogen, Islamist militants to a lesser or greater extent willingly decide to play an active role of some kind.

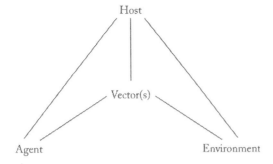

1.2 The Epidemic Model

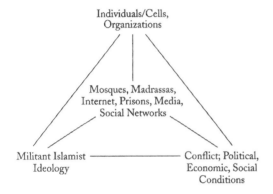

1.3 The Epidemic Model Applied to Islamist Militancy

Yet their actions are clearly driven by a core set of ideas and beliefs—an ideology—that has an "infectious" appeal. In this and other respects, Islamist militancy can be seen as having epidemic-like qualities. It, too, therefore, can be deconstructed using the classic epidemic model, as shown in figure 1.3.

Thus, with the model so applied, the agent is Islamist militant ideology. Specifically, two primary strains can be identified: (1) a transnational Salafist/ jihadist ideology as espoused by al Qaeda[8] and (2) a nationalist/ insurgent Islamist militant ideology as espoused by groups such as Hezbollah, Hamas, and some of the militant Kashmiri groups. Each ideological strain is characterized by a specific set of underlying assumptions, motivations, and goals.

The host is the group or person "infected" by the agent. More specifically, the host is a group or individual who becomes to a lesser or greater
extent an adherent of militant Islamist ideology. As defined, Islamist
militants are those who employ or espouse the use of violence in pursuit
of political goals.

The environment comprises key factors specific to the Muslim world
that promote exposure to Islamist militancy—conflict, political repression, economic stagnation, and social alienation being the leading
influences. Vectors in this case are a variety of known conduits that are
used to propagate the ideology and associated action agendas, such as
mosques, prisons, madrassas, the Internet, satellite television, and dia-
sporic networks.

It is important to understand that the epidemic model of Islamist
militancy acknowledges that the vast majority of Muslims find the core
elements of Islamist militant ideology both aberrant and abhorrent. In
this respect, they are effectively "immune" to its appeal. However, some
unknown, yet critical, proportion of the population is clearly "susceptible" to not only becoming an adherent of the ideology but being actively
motivated by it.

Several policy-relevant benefits accrue from conceiving of Islamist
militancy in this fashion. First, it captures the key elements of the challenge in a *systemic* manner rather than in the disaggregated, uncon-
nected way that so often bedevils analysis and understanding. Second, it
is a *dynamic* model that acknowledges that the phenomenon is not static
but constantly evolving with the emergence of new strains, new hosts,
new vectors, and changing environmental conditions. Third, it provides
insights into how Islamist militancy may evolve in the future.

However, unlike with an outbreak of disease, in which those infected
typically (though not always) are motivated to report their condition
to seek treatment, the size and spread of Islamist militancy are clearly
more difficult to assess. A combination of indicators (e.g., the number of
attacks conducted or thwarted and militants killed or incarcerated, the
influence of jihadist Web sites, the dissemination of training materials)
suggests that the phenomenon is expanding as well as mutating in the
ways indicated earlier. Surveys within the Muslim world, of people's attitudes toward the United States and the West more generally, would also
suggest that the pool of "susceptibles"—those at risk of becoming Islamist

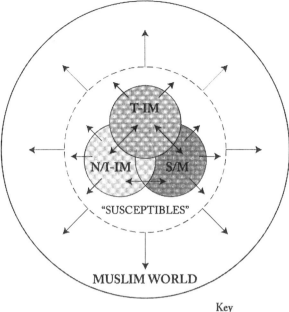

1.4 Growth of the "Epidemic"

Key
T-IM = transnational Islamist militants
N/I-IM = nationalist/insurgent Islamist militants
S/M = support/mobilization networks

militants—is large and expanding in certain countries. Figure 1.4 depicts the overall growth of Islamist militancy.

The Counter-epidemic Approach

Faced with the outbreak of an infectious disease, public health officials typically employ a three-pronged strategy to counter the threat.

First, *contain* the most threatening outbreaks and prevent them from gaining enough mass and momentum to overwhelm public health responders and threaten public order. Standard measures include quarantining specific areas to contain the movement of infectious individuals, eliminating or decontaminating identifiable vectors of transmission, and, if an antidote exists, treating and rehabilitating individuals who have succumbed to the disease. Containing and contracting the number of infectives can effectively eradicate the pathogen, though such a success is rare, as indicated earlier.

Second, *protect* those who are most vulnerable or susceptible to the disease (high-risk groups) as well as those who are most critical to a functioning society (high-value groups). The most effective countermeasure is selective or targeted immunization programs. Interestingly, not everyone needs to be inoculated in order to achieve what is known as "herd immunity"—essentially, the level at which the probability of an infected person being in contact with a nonimmunized person is very low, if not zero. If an effective vaccine is not available, other protective strategies are employed, including encouraging "safe practices" through public education to reduce the probability of exposure and the rate of new infection.

Third, *remedy* the environmental conditions that fostered the emergence of the disease in specific areas and its subsequent spread. Many types of interventions are conceivable, from the local to the global, depending on the nature of the threat.

Adapting the same basic strategic imperatives of a counter-epidemic campaign to the threat posed by Islamist militancy would immediately translate into the following operational priorities:

» Containing and contracting the activities of the most "virulent" Islamist militant organizations—the transnational jihadist groups with global reach and apocalyptic agendas—as well as those who could gain a meaningful operational presence in areas of significant strategic interest. These areas would include, most notably, Iraq, Pakistan, Afghanistan, Saudi Arabia, Egypt, Palestine, the Caucasus, and the Muslim diaspora communities of Western Europe as well as areas of key global financial and economic infrastructure assets.

» Protecting the high-risk and high-value communities of the Muslim world. According to open-source (unclassified) accounts, a disproportionate number of the officers and foot soldiers in the transnational jihadist cause come from a few countries—Saudi Arabia, Egypt, Morocco, Algeria, Yemen, Pakistan—and from the European diaspora communities. The high-value communities consist of the educational, religious, political, and security sectors of countries where Islamist militant organizations could make the greatest inroads and the growing number of transnational cultural, business, and media networks that affect the lives of many millions of Muslims throughout the larger *ummah* (Islamic community).

» Remedying the key environmental factors that foster Islamist militancy. The most important would appear to be the ongoing conflicts or insurgencies involving Muslims and non-Muslims that help validate the central jihadist

argument that Islam is under attack, and that also serve as recruiting mag-
nets and training grounds—notably, in Iraq, Palestine, Kashmir, Afghanistan,
Chechnya, and several smaller conflicts in Central and Southeast Asia.
Social alienation within the European diaspora communities and public cor-
ruption, political repression, and economic stagnation in key areas of the
Muslim world are widely viewed as additional factors.

These strategic imperatives can be further translated into specific containment, protective, and remedial programs or initiatives that, again,
draw on the principles and practices of a counter-epidemic campaign.

Containment Measures

In addition to limiting the operational reach and capabilities of the most
threatening Islamist militant organizations by using standard counterterrorism measures and discrete special intelligence and military operations, containment initiatives would extend to placing greater emphasis
on disrupting and restricting the untrammeled use of key vectors—the
Internet, satellite TV, prisons, schools, mosques, and so on—by Islamist
militant organizations. Some vectors can be physically shut down, others
"decontaminated" of unwanted infectious agents.[9] Containment measures appear to be a largely haphazard, after-the-fact effort at this time
rather than a systematically planned, internationally executed campaign.

Because of the practical limits to such efforts in an open society,
greater attention should also be given to nurturing and propagating
what can be termed an "ideological antidote" to the key tenets of Islamist
militant ideology. This can involve a broad-gauge campaign to denounce
and delegitimize jihadist propaganda and practices such as beheadings
and the killing of innocent civilians, including fellow Muslims, as well as
more discrete efforts aimed toward a specific group or community. The
former includes mobilizing moderate religious figures to issue fatwas
condemning the ideology and tactics used as a perversion of Islam and
encouraging key opinion makers, cultural leaders, and mass-media figures to do the same.[10] Such efforts have been made but apparently not in
an extensive or concerted way.[11] More targeted activities include exploiting the ideological contradictions or schisms within the transnational
jihadist movement in order to foment internal dissension and possible

defections. There are reports, for example, of successful counter-ideological efforts in Yemen that in turn yielded operational success in rolling up a local al Qaeda network.[12]

Although many Islamist militants are beyond such intellectual suasion—essentially the equivalent of treatment and rehabilitation in health care—this may not be the case with some groups and organizations. Local national-insurgent movements, in particular, may be susceptible to a "rehabilitative" process in much the way that other terrorist groups have been led to abandon armed struggle. The evolving role of groups such as Hamas and Hezbollah, for example, suggests the possibility of their integration into their respective political systems. The provision of amnesty to insurgents willing to lay down arms, as in Afghanistan, constitutes another element of rehabilitation. And in Iraq, reports suggested a growing rift between the nationalist Iraqi elements of the insurgency and foreign jihadists, in part as a result of the latter's indiscriminate targeting of civilians.[13]

Protective Measures

Whereas containment measures are directed primarily at those already infected, protective measures are aimed at those who are most at risk and those who play important societal functions. It is conceivable that with better understanding of why certain groups and individuals become first sympathetic to, then supportive of, and finally actively engaged in Islamist militant causes, targeted programs that effectively immunize at-risk groups could be designed. There are many cases in which key populations have been targeted in ways designed to turn off their receptiveness to specific ideas, messages, and unhealthy or antisocial practices, including through appeals to common sense, personal safety, peer-group standing, religious edicts and societal norms, among other approaches. In some cases, the tactics used are not unlike real vaccination programs that work on the principle of exposing uninfected populations to a weakened or attenuated version of the virus so that the body learns to identify and reject the real thing. Political campaigns, for example, often expose key undecided voters to the arguments of opposing candidates, in some cases to ridicule the candidates but more often to "arm" voters with convincing reasons to be skeptical when they hear the same arguments from those candidates.[14]

Similar public programs aimed at undermining the appeal of militant Islamist ideology could be designed and implemented in many different arenas, from schools to mosques to mass-media outlets. Unless they are undertaken in the Muslim communities of Western Europe, however, these are clearly not initiatives that the United States (and the West more generally) should lead or be openly associated with, although Western states can prod allies and partners in the Muslim world and provide discreet assistance.

Such "ideological immunization" efforts aimed at high-risk communities should not just provide a negative image of militant Islamism. Ideally, they should also offer a positive and compelling alternative vision for the future. Indeed, efforts to undermine militant Islamism and provide a positive counter-ideology can be mutually reinforcing. Again, the same arenas and conduits—schools, mosques, mass-media outlets—have a critical role to play, and thus efforts designed to mobilize and strengthen moderate voices in these sectors should be an indispensable component of the overall effort.[15]

Remedial Measures

Many of the previous initiatives will be harder to accomplish or will likely fail if parallel efforts are not also taken to remedy some of the key environmental conditions that promote Islamist militancy in the Muslim world. For reasons discussed earlier, an intensified effort should be made to resolve or at least tamp down the violent conflicts that have a particularly strong resonance within the Muslim world. Indeed, successful conflict management and prevention strategies will play a key role in impeding the spread of Islamist militancy. Besides reducing the direct role of the violent conflict in jihadist recruitment and training, conflict resolution efforts will help invalidate jihadist propaganda and buttress moderate support.

The implementation of political reforms focused on good governance, particularly greater transparency, accountability, and the rule of law, will also play a key role in neutralizing Islamist militant ideology that calls for the overthrow of corrupt regimes. Likewise, greater civil liberties, including broader freedoms of assembly and expression as well as the freedom to form political parties and other associations, will help

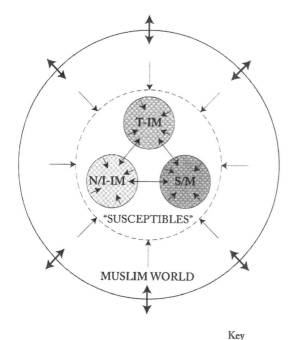

Key
T-IM = transnational Islamist militants
N/I-IM = nationalist/insurgent Islamist militants
S/M = support/mobilization networks

1.5 Countering the "Epidemic"

level the political playing field and allow "healthy" outlets for dissent. Particular emphasis should be placed on institution building so as to prevent democratic gains from being undermined by autocratic regimes or exploited by nondemocratic opposition forces. Facilitating the political participation of peaceful, moderate Islamists can also help develop an effective counterweight to Islamist militants and their violent tactics.

The implementation of economic reforms designed to spur growth and bolster job creation will likewise help ease popular disaffection, particularly among the region's disproportionately young population. In addition, economic reforms that create an environment that is more appealing to foreign investors will help the Muslim world integrate more effectively into the broader global economic system and help bridge the gap in relative performance between the Muslim world, particularly the Arab world, and the global economy.

The combined effect of these containment, protective, and remedial measures will be to reverse over time the negative trends discussed ear-

PAUL B. STARES AND MONA YACOUBIAN

lier. As figure 1.5 depicts, the effect will be to divide, isolate, and weaken Islamist militant organizations and marginalize their operational impact. The pool of susceptibles will also shrink in relation to the rest of the Muslim world, which, through the various remedial efforts, will become a more "healthy" and integrated part of the larger, globalizing world.

As with a global health campaign, success in countering the challenge of Islamist militancy depends on a sustained commitment over many years, if not decades, by a broad coalition of like-minded states acting in partnership with a multitude of nongovernmental actors. Simply stated, there is no single or easy cure.

Concluding Observations

The counter-epidemic approach to meeting the challenge of Islamist militancy follows in fundamental respects the basic tenets of effective conflict prevention and management. These tenets can be summarized as follows using common admonitions from the world of public health care:

> » *Prevention is better than cure.* Reducing the momentum of a conflict, especially after passions have become inflamed and blood spilt, is clearly more difficult than taking early preventive measures to forestall violence; positions harden, options narrow, and the costs rise. Early warning and early response can therefore make all the difference.
>
> » *Diagnose before treating.* Knowing thy ailment is just as important as knowing thy enemy. While it doesn't guarantee success, clearly understanding the source(s) and dynamics of a conflict before taking action obviously improves the chances of applying the right tools in the right place with the right outcomes.
>
> » *Do no harm.* The Hippocratic Oath is no less relevant to conflict management. As countless examples attest, poorly timed or calibrated interventions can make a problem worse, not better. Knowing what to do and when to do it in conflict management is as much an art as a science, but again, experience provides a rich set of guidelines, particularly when it comes to balancing incentives and disincentives, force with diplomacy, and so on.
>
> » *Address the source, not the symptoms;* Resolving the root cause of a conflict typically raises the bar in terms of what is required to secure peace, but as many long-festering disputes attest, the Band-Aid approach to conflict

management at best delays and in many instances complicates the task of finding a sustainable solution.

» *Palliate when you cannot cure.* Sometimes, a solution is beyond practical reach. Just as some diseases are—for the time being, at least—incurable, some conflicts become, for all intents and purposes, intractable. Under such circumstances, the best that can be achieved is to limit the consequences and not make a bad situation worse.

As indicated at the outset, however, the task of conflict prevention and management must adapt to the emerging realities of the twenty-first century. As a consequence of the forces of globalization, the world has clearly become a smaller, more interconnected place. Threats to international peace and stability that may have previously been considered distant and inconsequential now resonate more widely, more quickly, and with greater impact. For similar reasons, nonstate actors can now wield unprecedented power for good and bad while also having much greater latitude to operate across borders—again, with positive and negative consequences, as al Qaeda and numerous warlords around the world have demonstrated.

At the same time, states seeking to prevent and manage conflict, whether it be within their borders or in areas both adjacent and distant, find themselves in a changed operating environment. In addition to the interdependencies of a globalizing world, emerging legal rules and norms affect their freedom much more than was previously the case. Their actions, furthermore, are subject to greater scrutiny and accountability by virtue of not only the constant 24/7 gaze of the global media but also an expanding network of intergovernmental and nongovernmental organizations (NGOs).

As a consequence of these new realities, states can rarely, if ever, address threats to peace and stability as singular actors. The task is likely to be too big to solve alone, while important advantages—not least in terms of generating international legitimacy—can be derived from acting collectively. This imperative to cooperate may seem too high a price to pay to those concerned about national sovereignty, but such concerns are arguably becoming redundant in an increasingly interdependent world if they haven't already become so. Indeed, giving up some de jure sovereignty may be the only way for states to regain some de facto sovereignty, especially when it comes to nonstate-based threats such as transnational terrorism.

The growing imperative for international cooperation is matched by the comparable need for states to partner with nongovernmental actors and civil society in general. The benefits are mutual. States need the cooperation of NGOs in order to manage those who would exploit the business and commercial sectors, among others, for nefarious ends, and NGOs likewise need the support of governments if they are to operate effectively and relatively freely. Again, such partnerships can confer legitimacy on both sides.

Finally, states must adapt their internal political and bureaucratic structures and processes to these new imperatives. What were largely vestiges of the Cold War and earlier eras have to be reformed or replaced with new mechanisms for governmental decision making, coordination, and implementation. Without such changes, effective conflict prevention and management will only become more difficult to achieve.

NOTES

1   See National Commission on Terrorist Attacks, *The 9/11 Commission Report: Final Report of the National Commission on Terrorist Attacks upon the United States* (New York: W. W. Norton, 2004), 362n3.

2   We recognize, therefore, that there are also peaceful Islamist organizations, including legal Islamist political parties such as the Party for Justice and Development in Morocco and charitable organizations such as the Red Crescent.

3   See, for example, David J. Kilcullen, "Countering Global Insurgency," *Journal of Strategic Studies* 28, no. 4 (August 2005): 597–617; and Bruce Hoffman, testimony to the House Armed Services Committee, Subcommittee on Terrorism, Unconventional Threats and Capabilities, 109th Cong., 2nd sess., February 16, 2006.

4   See, for example, Malcolm Gladwell, *The Tipping Point: How Little Things Can Make a Big Difference* (Boston: First Back Bay, 2002); Joshua M. Epstein, "Modeling Civil Violence: An Agent-Based Computational Approach," *Proceedings of the National Academy of Sciences* vol. 99, suppl. 3 (May 14, 2003): 7243–50; Luis M. A. Bettancourt et al., "The Power of a Good Idea: Quantitative Models," Santa Fe Institute Working Paper, February 6 (Santa Fe, N.Mex.: Santa Fe Institute, 2005).

5   For example, Richard N. Haass, former director of policy planning, U.S.

State Department, went further in drawing the analogy in a major speech: "The challenge of terrorism is . . . akin to fighting a virus in that we can accomplish a great deal but not eradicate the problem. We can take steps to prevent it, protect ourselves from it, and when an attack occurs, quarantine it, minimize the damage it inflicts, and attack it with all our power." Richard N. Haass, Speech to the Council on Foreign Relations, New York, October 15, 2001. Likewise, France's top counterterrorism official, Judge Jean-Louis Bruguière, has often compared the terrorist threat posed by groups such as al Qaeda to a mutating virus. See, for example, "Al Qaeda's New Front," *Frontline*, October 12, 2004, PBS, http:www.pbs.org/wgbh/pages/frontline/shows/front/map/bruguiere.html.

6   Numerous examples of "tipping points" exist in nearly every realm of life, from fashion to politics. The reversal of New York City's burgeoning crime wave in the 1980s stands as a classic example of identifying and successfully exploiting a tipping point. In that case, the police embarked on a strategy of cracking down on relatively minor "quality of life" crimes. They went after panhandlers and subway fare cheats as well as made a concerted effort to remove the graffiti from subway cars and ensure that they stay clean. These relatively minor measures constituted a key tipping point that apparently contributed to a significant downturn in serious crime.

7   We consulted two key references for this section: B. Burt Gerstman, *Epidemiology Kept Simple: An Introduction to Traditional and Modern Epidemiology* (Hoboken, N.J.: Wiley Liss, 2003); and Leon Gordis, *Epidemiology*, 3rd ed. (Philadelphia: Elsevier Saunders, 2004).

8   The modern Salafi movement traces its roots to the nineteenth-century Egyptian religious figure Muhammad Abduh and his disciple Rashid Rida, who denounced the innovations and schisms (notably the Sunni-Shiite divide) within the Muslim community as perversions of Islam. Salafists demand a return to the pure form of Islam as practiced by the Prophet Muhammad and his immediate successors. Over the past two centuries, the Salafi movement has evolved, split, and adapted to differing circumstances throughout the Muslim world. Salafists do not necessarily call for the use of violence; some focus almost exclusively on social behavior, advocating an ultraconservative moral code to direct dress and other social practices. However, a violent, extremist branch of the movement combines the missionary zeal associated with the call to purge Islam of its impure elements with the violent anti-Western extremism incubated among jihadists in Afghanistan in the 1980s and 1990s. Sources on the Salafist jihadist ideology include Quintan Wiktorowicz, "The New Global Threat: Transnational Salafis and Jihad," *Middle East Policy* 8, no. 4 (December 2001): 18–38; Christopher M. Blanchard, *Al*

Qaeda: Statements and Evolving Ideology, CRS Report for Congress, February 4 (Washington, D.C.: U.S. Department of State, 2005); Anonymous, *Through Our Enemies' Eyes: Osama Bin Laden, Radical Islam, and the Future of America* (Washington, D.C.: Brassey's, 2002); and Gilles Kepel, *The War for Muslim Minds* (Cambridge, Mass.: Harvard University Press, 2004).

9   For example, in February 2005, London's Finsbury Park mosque, once a bastion of radicalism, was reclaimed. A new board of directors ousted the mosque's radical cleric, Abu Hamza al-Masri, and literally changed the locks. See Lizette Alvarez, "Britain's Mainstream Muslims Find Voice," *New York Times*, March 6, 2005. Similarly, measures must be taken within prison systems to curtail and ultimately cease recruitment. For specific recommendations, see Ian Cuthbertson, "Prisons and the Education of Terrorists," *World Policy Journal* 21, no. 3 (Fall 2004): 20.

10 Alvarez, "Britain's Mainstream Muslims Find Voice." Mainstream Muslims in Britain have also taken steps to isolate Islamist militants and strengthen ties between moderates and the British establishment.

11 See David E. Kaplan, "Hearts, Minds, and Dollars," *U.S. News and World Report*, April 25, 2005.

12 See James Brandon, "Koranic Duel Eases Terror," *Christian Science Monitor*, February 4, 2005.

13 Sabrina Tavernise, "Marines See Signs Iraq Rebels Are Battling Foreign Fighters," *New York Times*, June 21, 2005.

14 See Matt Bai, "The Framing Wars," *New York Times Magazine*, July 12, 2005. See also Bettancourt et al., "The Power of a Good Idea," 10.

15 Jordan, for example, has undertaken a broad curriculum review that emphasizes more moderate and progressive interpretations of Islam. See Hassan M. Fattah, "Jordan Is Preparing to Tone Down the Islamic Bombast in Textbooks," *New York Times*, June 12, 2005. A number of European governments are also exploring options for having greater influence over the training of imams who preach in European mosques. See Elaine Sciolino, "Europe Struggling to Train New Breed of Muslim Clerics," *New York Times*, October 18, 2004.

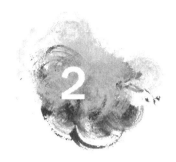

EPIDEMIC INTELLIGENCE

Toward a Genealogy of Global Health Security

Andrew Lakoff

T his chapter considers how public health authorities respond to the threat of contagion in a period of widespread concern about newly emerging diseases that can spread rapidly across borders and wreak havoc on both global health and global economies. The goal of the chapter is neither to assess the likelihood of such an epidemic nor to evaluate whether or not officials and experts are adequately responding to this threat. Rather, the chapter examines the conditions of possibility for thinking about infectious disease in a certain way. How, in other words, have experts and officials come to envision the contemporary problem of contagion, and what responses have they proposed? Specifically, the chapter contrasts two ways of taking up the problem of contagious disease at a global scale: "global health security" and "humanitarian biomedicine."

Global health security focuses on emerging infectious diseases— whether naturally occurring or man-made—that are seen to threaten wealthy countries and to emanate from poorer parts of the world. Its exemplary pathogens include Ebola, SARS, and highly virulent influenza, but what is crucial is that this way of envisioning disease is oriented toward outbreaks that *have not yet occurred*—and may never occur. For this reason, global health security develops techniques of preparedness for events of incalculable probability that could have catastrophic political, economic and health consequences. Its practitioners seek to create a real-time, global disease surveillance mechanism that can provide early warning of potential outbreaks in developing countries and to link such detection to immediate methods of response that will protect against their spread to the rest of the world. In order to build this preparedness system, global health security initiatives draw together various organizations, including multilateral health agencies, national disease control institutes, and collaborative reference laboratories, and assemble diverse technical elements such as disease surveillance methods, emergency operations centers, and vaccine distribution systems.

45

Humanitarian biomedicine, in contrast, targets diseases that afflict populations in the poorer parts of the world, such as malaria, tuberculosis, and HIV/AIDS. Its problematic is one of alleviating human suffering, regardless of national boundaries or social groupings. Such intervention is called for where public health infrastructure at the nation-state level is in poor condition or is nonexistent. Humanitarian biomedicine tends to develop linkages outside the state—between nongovernmental organizations, activists, scientific researchers, and local health workers. Its target of intervention is not a collectivity conceived as a national population but rather individual human lives. Advocates of humanitarian biomedicine seek to bring advanced diagnostic and pharmaceutical interventions to those in need, a project that involves both providing access to existing medical technologies and spurring the development of new medications that address neglected diseases. Whereas global health security develops prophylaxis against potential future threats at home, humanitarian biomedicine invests resources in mitigating current suffering in other places.

Governing Pathogens

A recent case illustrates some of the tensions that arise at the intersection of these two different ways of understanding and intervening in infectious disease. In an opinion piece published in the *Washington Post* on

August 10, 2008, diplomat Richard Holbrooke and science journalist Laurie Garrett mounted a sharp attack on what they called "viral sovereignty." By this term, the authors referred to the "extremely dangerous" idea that sovereign states could exercise ownership rights over samples of viruses found in their territory. Specifically, Holbrooke and Garrett were incensed by the Indonesian government's refusal to share samples of Avian Influenza A (H5N1) with the Global Influenza Surveillance Network (GISN) of the World Health Organization (WHO). For more than fifty years, this network had collected samples of flu viruses from around the world and used them to determine the composition of yearly flu vaccines. More recently, the network had monitored the transformations of avian influenza viruses as a means of assessing the risk of a deadly global pandemic.[1] International health experts feared that the new strain of H5N1, which had already proved highly virulent, would mutate to become easily transmissible among humans, in which case a worldwide calamity could be at hand. GISN thus served as a global early-warning system enabling experts to track genetic changes in the virus that could lead to a catastrophic disease event.

As the country where the highest number of human cases of avian influenza had so far been reported, Indonesia was a potential epicenter of such an outbreak. For this reason, the country's decision to withhold samples of the virus undermined GISN's function as a global early-warning system. From Holbrooke and Garrett's vantage point, Indonesia's action posed a significant threat to global health security. "In this age of globalization," they wrote, "failure to make viral samples open-source risks allowing the emergence of a new strain of influenza that could go unnoticed until it is capable of exacting the sort of toll taken by the pandemic that killed tens of millions in 1918." According to Garrett and Holbrooke, Indonesia had not only a moral but also a legal obligation to share its viruses with the World Health Organization. They argued that the country's action was a violation of the newly revised International Health Regulations (IHR), which held the status of an international treaty for WHO member states.

The opinion piece suggested that the rational and beneficent WHO technocracy was faced with antiscientific demagoguery that threatened global health. Holbrooke and Garrett painted a picture of the Indonesian health minister, Siti Fadilah Supari, as an irrational populist who sought to make domestic political gains through unfounded attacks on the United States and the international health community. Indonesia was apparently withholding these virus samples based on the "dangerous folly" of thinking that the materials should be protected through the same legal mechanism that the United Nations Food and Agriculture Organization uses to guarantee poor countries' rights of ownership to indigenous agricultural resources, the Convention on Biological Diversity. Further, Holbrooke and Garrett rebuked Supari for her "outlandish claims" that the U.S. government was planning to use Indonesia's H5N1 samples to design biological warfare agents, echoing U.S. Secretary of Defense Robert Gates's reaction upon hearing this accusation during a visit to Jakarta: "the nuttiest idea I've ever heard."[2]

The controversy over influenza virus sharing was, it turned out, somewhat more complicated than Holbrooke and Garrett allowed. Beginning in late 2006, at Supari's behest, the Indonesian Health Ministry had stopped sharing isolates of H5N1 found in patients who had died of avian influenza with the Global Influenza Surveillance Network. The source of Supari's ire was the discovery that an Australian pharmaceutical company had developed a patented vaccine for avian flu using an Indonesian strain of the virus—a vaccine that most Indonesians would not be able to afford in the event of a deadly pandemic. More generally, given the limited number of vaccine doses that could be produced in time to manage such a pandemic—estimates were in the 500 million range—experts acknowledged that developing countries would have little access to such a vaccine. In other words, while Indonesia had been delivering virus samples to WHO as part of a collective early-warning mechanism (i.e., GISN), its people would not be beneficiaries of the biomedical response apparatus constructed to prepare for a deadly global outbreak. For the Indonesian health minister, this situation indicated a dark "conspiracy between superpower nations and global organizations."

While less suspicious than Supari of U.S. and WHO intentions, a number of Western journalists and scientists were sympathetic to the Indonesian position on the grounds of equity in the global distribution of necessary medicines. A *Time* magazine article noted that "they had a point; poor developing nations are often priced out of needed medicines, and they're likely to be last in line for vaccine during a pandemic."[3] An editorial in the *Lancet* argued that "to ensure global health security, countries have to protect the wellbeing not only of their own patients but also those of fellow nations."[4] Anxious to ensure the functioning of its influenza surveillance apparatus, WHO was willing to strike a bargain: at a World Health Assembly meeting in 2007, members agreed to explore ways of helping poorer countries build vaccine production capacity. But the financial and technical details of how such a system would function were opaque, and the issue remained unresolved. In October 2008, as Indonesia continued to withhold the vast majority of its avian influenza samples from GISN, Agence France-Presse reported that "Supari does appear to be vindicated by a flood of patents being lodged on the samples of H5N1 that have made it out of Indonesia, with companies in developed countries claiming ownership over viral DNA taken from sick Indonesians."[5] The Australian company CSL Limited acknowledged that it had used Indonesian bird flu strains to develop a trial vaccine but insisted that it had no obligation to compensate Indonesia or guarantee access to the vaccine. Unlike the data generated by GISN, vaccines themselves were not open-source.

One aspect of Holbrooke and Garrett's critique, their accusation that Indonesia was in violation of the revised International Health Regulations, deserves closer examination. The IHR system, dating from the 1851 International Sanitary Law, defines states' mutual obligations in the event of an outbreak of a dangerous communicable disease. Historically, its function has been to guarantee the continued flow of global commodities during such outbreaks, ensuring that countries do not take overly restrictive measures in response to the threat of infection. The H5N1 virus-sharing controversy unfolded just after a major revision of these regulations. According to legal scholar David Fidler, the 2005 IHR revision was "one of the most radical and far-reaching changes in international law on public health since the beginning of international health co-operation in the mid-nineteenth century."[6]

For the purposes of this chapter, the revised International Health Regulations are best understood as a significant element in an emerging apparatus of global disease surveillance and response—what the World Health Organization calls "global public health security." The regulations instituted a new set of legal obligations under which nation-states had to accept external intervention in a world seen as threatened by ominous pathogens circulating ever more rapidly. A key provision expanded the list of the diseases that were subject to international regulation and potential intervention beyond the classic infections of the nineteenth century—cholera, yellow fever, and plague. With the revision, any disease outbreak that could be classified as a "public health emergency of international concern"—such as SARS or an easily transmissible form of H_5N_1—would be covered by the regulations. International law experts saw the virus-sharing controversy as an early test of how well the revised regulations would function.

According to the new regulations, IHR signatories were required to provide WHO with public health information about events that might constitute a public health emergency of international concern (PHEIC).[7] In the case of the Indonesian virus-sharing controversy, the central legal question was whether biological samples were instances of such public health information. Plausible arguments could be made on both sides. At the May 2007 meeting of the World Health Assembly, WHO director-general Margaret Chan claimed, "countries that did not share avian influenza virus would fail the IHR."[8] The U.S. delegation agreed: "All nations have a responsibility under the revised IHRs to share data and virus samples on a timely basis and without preconditions."[9] Thus, the United States argued, "our view is that withholding influenza viruses from GISN greatly threatens global public health and will violate the legal obligations we have all agreed to undertake through our adherence to IHRs."[10] However, the relevance of the revised International Health Regulations to the specific issue of virus sharing was ambiguous: the new regulations explicitly referred only to a requirement to share public health *information*, such as case reports and fatality rates, and some observers argued that biological materials such as virus samples were distinct from such information.[11]

In any case, the Indonesian health ministry's response came from outside the legal framework of the International Health Regulations. Supari argued that the global virus-sharing system was ethically compromised and in need of reform. "We want to change the global virus sharing mechanism to be fair, transparent and equitable," she said in an interview defending the government's decision to withhold the virus.[12] "What we mean by fair is that any virus sharing should be accompanied by benefits derived from the shared virus, and these benefits should be coming from the vaccine producing countries." Supari was speaking from within a different problematic than that of WHO's framework of "global public health security," the strategy that the revised regulations were designed to serve. In speaking of sharing benefits, Supari was invoking a mechanism intended to encourage development, the Convention on Biological Diversity, in order to ground a rhetoric of national sovereignty that ran counter to the transnational authority of WHO, but her attack on the high price of patented vaccines also resonated with demands for equal access to life-saving medicines coming out of the humanitarian biomedicine movement.

A technical and political system designed to prepare for potentially catastrophic disease outbreaks was facing a very different demand: a call for access to essential medicines based on a political vision of global equity (see fig. 2.1). The potential for a deadly outbreak of avian influenza had led to an encounter between two different ways of conceptualizing the problem of global disease outbreaks, one that was taking place in the absence of an actual health emergency. At stake was the issue of not only how best to respond to a global outbreak of H5N1 but, more broadly, how to define the political obligation to care for the population's health in a globalizing world in which the capacity of national public health authorities to protect citizens' well-being was increasingly in question.

Assembling Global Health

Each of these ways of managing global contagion can be seen as a response to a crisis of existing, nation-state–based systems of public health. From the vantage of global health security, this crisis comes from the recognition that existing national public health systems are inadequate to prepare for the potentially catastrophic threat of emerging infectious diseases. Such diseases outstrip the capabilities of modern public health systems that were designed to manage known diseases that occur with regularity in a national population. For humanitarian biomedicine, in contrast, the crisis comes from the failure of nation-states to provide adequate health infrastructure that would lessen the burden of treatable, but still deadly maladies in poor countries: it is a political and technical failure rather than the result of disease emergence per se. For humanitarian biomedicine, especially in the context of states in which public health

	Global Health Security	Humanitarian Biomedicine
Type of threat	Emerging infectious diseases that threaten wealthy countries	Neglected diseases that afflict poor countries
Source of pathogenicity	Social and ecological transformations linked to globalization	Failure of development; lack of access to health care
Organizations and actors	National and international health agencies; technocrats	NGOs, philanthropies, activists
Technopolitical interventions	Global disease surveillance; building response capacity; rapidly develop biomedical interventions to manage novel pathogens	Provide access to essential medicines; drug and vaccine research and development for diseases of the poor
Target of Intervention	National public health infrastructures	Suffering individuals
Ethical stance	Self-protection	Common humanity

2.1 Two Ways of Envisioning Disease Threats

infrastructure has deteriorated, human suffering demands urgent and immediate responses outside the framework of state sovereignty.

Despite their differences, each of these ways of seeing infectious disease has borrowed certain aspects of earlier public health formations, adapting them for new uses in the post–Cold War era. The first public health systems in Europe and North America were built in the mid-to-late nineteenth century in response to social pathologies linked to industrialization in urban centers.[13] For these systems, the object of knowledge and intervention was the population: its rates of death and disease, cycles of scarcity, and endemic levels of mortality. Early public health advocates uncovered patterns of disease incidence linked to living conditions that could be reduced through technical interventions.[14] Statistical knowledge, generated in fields such as epidemiology and demography, made these collective regularities visible. Public health advocates sought to know and manage such regularities, to decrease mortality and increase longevity—to "optimize a state of life," as Michel Foucault put it.[15]

For this early form of public health, the rational design of interventions required analysis of historical patterns of disease in a given population. For example, as historian George Rosen has shown, nineteenth-century British public health reformers carefully tracked the incidence of disease according to differential social locations in order to make the argument that "health was affected for better or worse by the state of the physical or social environment."[16] Such knowledge was cumulative and calculative. Reformers gathered and analyzed vital statistics—rates of birth, death, and illness among various classes—in order to demonstrate the economic rationality of disease prevention measures such as the provision of clean water or the removal of waste from streets.[17] If this initial mode of public health intervention emphasized social conditions such as sanitation, nutrition, and occupational safety, a subsequent iteration of public health narrowed its focus to the level of the pathogen. The rise of bacteriology in the late nineteenth century led to the systematic practice of mass vaccination against infectious disease. But again, for these early forms of public health, making rational interventions required statistical knowledge about the historical pattern of disease incidence in a specific population.[18]

Cold War–era international health efforts, as exemplified by the World Health Organization after its founding in 1948, had two main currents: disease eradication and primary health care.[19] The major international disease eradication efforts were the WHO-led malaria campaign begun in 1955 and abandoned by the early 1970s and the more successful smallpox eradication campaign, again led by WHO, completed in 1977. The WHO-led disease eradication initiatives were international, rather than "global," in that they required coordination between WHO and national public health services. The other main current of Cold War–era international health, primary health care, articulated health as a basic human right linked to social and economic development.[20] Again, this vision was international rather than global: for advocates of primary health care efforts, a functioning nation-state apparatus was central to the delivery of basic primary care, and so state-based development efforts were critical to the improvement of the population's health.

By the early 1990s, the primary health care model linked to the developmental state was in crisis. Funding dried up for primary health care schemes in the context of privatizing reforms of national health systems led by the World Bank. WHO shifted its energies toward vertically integrated public-private partnerships that focused on managing specific diseases, such as HIV/AIDS and tuberculosis, rather than on developing local health infrastructures. As a group of public health historians has recently suggested, competition between the World Health Organization and the World Bank over the field of primary care was one motivation for WHO's move toward such public-private global health initiatives.[21] The Bill & Melinda Gates Foundation also played a key early role in this shift, funding $1.7 billion worth of projects from 1998 to 2000. The Gates Foundation was then joined in this type of disease-focused initiative by other donor-funded institutions, such as the Global Fund to Fight AIDS, Tuberculosis and Malaria and the Clinton Global Initiative.

These contemporary projects for managing infectious disease on a global scale take up aspects of earlier public health programs but adapt them to a different set of circumstances. Global health security seeks to direct certain elements of existing national health systems toward its goal of early detection and rapid containment of emerging infections. Since its focus is on *potential* disease events, whose likelihood cannot be calculated using statistical methods, it develops techniques of imaginative enactment that model the impact of an outbreak. Global health security demands compliance from national governments in developing preparedness measures for potential outbreaks that threaten global catastrophe. In contrast, humanitarian biomedicine is concerned with existing diseases, but it functions outside the state apparatus; its object of concern is not the national population but suffering individuals irrespective of national borders. If a major ethical imperative for classical public health efforts was one of social solidarity, humanitarian biomedicine emphasizes common humanity.[22]

Global Health Security

A 2007 report from the World Health Organization, "A Safer Future: Global Public Health Security in the 21st Century," provided a summary of the objects and aims of global health security.[23] The report began by noting the success of traditional public health measures during the twentieth century in dealing with devastating infectious diseases such as cholera and smallpox, although in recent decades, it noted, there had been an alarming shift in the "delicate balance between humans and microbes."[24] A series of factors—including demographic changes, economic development, global travel and commerce, and conflict—had "heightened the risk of disease outbreaks," ranging from new infectious diseases such as HIV/AIDS and drug-resistant tuberculosis to food-borne pathogens and bioterrorist attacks.[25]

The WHO report proposed a strategic framework for responding to this new landscape of threats, which it called "global public health security." The framework emphasized an arena of global health that was distinct from the predominantly national organization of traditional public health. "In the globalized world of the 21st century," the report argued, simply stopping disease at national borders is not adequate. Nor was it sufficient to respond to diseases after they have become established in a population. Rather, it was necessary to prepare for unknown outbreaks in advance, something that could be achieved only "if there is immediate alert and response to disease outbreaks and other incidents that could spark epidemics or spread globally and if there are national systems in place for detection and response should such events occur across international borders."[26]

WHO's framework of "global public health security" was a culmination of two decades of increasing concern over the problematic of emerging infectious disease, which had initially been raised by a group of U.S.-based infectious disease experts in the late 1980s and early 1990s.[27] In 1989, Nobel Prize–winning molecular biologist Joshua Lederberg and virologist Stephen Morse hosted a major conference on the topic, which led to the landmark volume *Emerging Viruses*.[28] Lederberg and Morse shared an ecological vision of disease emergence as the result of environmental transformation combined with increased global circulation.[29] Participants in the 1989 conference warned of a dangerous intersection. On the one hand, there were a number of new disease threats, including novel viruses such as AIDS and Ebola, as well as drug-resistant strains of diseases such as tuberculosis and malaria. On the other hand, public health systems worldwide had begun to decay, beginning in the late 1960s, because of the assumption that infectious disease had been conquered. Moreover, the appearance of new infectious diseases could be expected to continue, due to a number of global processes such as increased travel, urbanization, civil wars and refugee crises, and ecological incursion. For these experts, the AIDS crisis heralded a dangerous future in which more deadly diseases were likely to emerge.

Over the ensuing years, alarm about emerging disease threats came from various quarters, including prominent organizations such as the Institute of Medicine, journalists such as Laurie Garrett, and writers such as Richard Preston.[30] For many health experts, the threat of emerging disease—especially when combined with weakening national public health systems—marked a troublesome reversal in the history of public health. At just the moment when it seemed that infectious disease was about to be conquered, and that the critical health problems of the industrialized world now centered on chronic disease, these experts warned, we were witnessing a return of the microbe.

It is worth emphasizing the generative character of the category of emerging infectious disease, which made it possible to bring AIDS into relation with a range of other diseases, including viral hemorrhagic fevers, West Nile virus, dengue, and drug-resistant strains of malaria and tuberculosis. The category also pointed toward the imperative to develop means of anticipatory response that could deal with a disparate set of disease threats. Initiatives that would later come to be associated with global health security were first proposed in response to this perceived need.

Practices of disease eradication that had been honed as part of Cold War international health were incorporated into proposed solutions to the problem of emerging disease. One contributor to *Emerging Viruses*, epidemiologist D. A. Henderson, had implemented techniques of disease surveillance in the 1960s and 1970s as director of the WHO Smallpox Eradication Program. For Henderson, the task was one not of prevention but of vigilant monitoring. In the report, he argues that novel pathogen emergence is inevitable, that "mutation and change are facts of nature, that the world is increasingly interdependent, and that human health and survival will be challenged, ad infinitum, by new and mutant microbes, with unpredictable pathophysiological manifestations."[31] As a result, "we are uncertain as to what we should keep under surveillance, or even what we should look for." What we need, he continued, is a system that can detect novelty: in the case of AIDS, such a detection system could have provided early warning of the new virus and made it possible to put in place measures to limit its spread. Henderson proposed a global system of disease surveillance units to be run by the Centers for Disease Control and Prevention (CDC) and located in peri-urban areas in major cities in the tropics, which could provide a "window on events in surrounding areas." Thus, techniques for managing contagious disease that had been developed in an earlier period of international health—surveillance, outbreak investigation, and containment—were brought to bear to address the newly articulated problem of emerging infectious disease.

Over the course of the 1990s, the emerging disease problematic was integrated into U.S. national security discussions. National security experts began to focus on bioterrorism as one of a number of asymmetric threats the nation faced in the wake of the Cold War, hypothesizing an association between rogue states, global terrorist organizations, and the proliferation of weapons of mass destruction.[32] Reports during the 1990s about Soviet and Iraqi bioweapons programs, along with Aum Shinrikyo's Tokyo subway attack in 1995, lent credibility to calls for biodefense measures focused on the threat of bioterrorism. Early advocates of such efforts, including infectious disease specialists such as Henderson and national security officials such as Richard Clarke, claimed that adequate preparation for a biological attack would require a massive infusion of resources into both biomedical research and public health response capacity.[33] More broadly, they argued, it would be necessary to incorporate the agencies and institutions of the life sciences and public health into the national security establishment. In the 1990s, Henderson and others connected the interest in emerging disease among international health specialists with the concern among national security officials about the rise of bioterrorism, suggesting that a global disease surveillance network could address both problems.

Epidemic Intelligence

Henderson's model of disease surveillance came out of his background at the Epidemic Intelligence Service based at the CDC.[34] The approach, developed in the 1950s, was one of "continued watchfulness over the distribution and trends of incidence through systematic consolidation and evaluation of morbidity and mortality data and other relevant data," as his mentor Alexander Langmuir put it.[35] Henderson used this method in tracking the global incidence of smallpox while he was director of the WHO eradication program. His proposed global network of surveillance centers and reference laboratories extended this approach to as yet unknown diseases, providing early warning for outbreaks of any kind, whether natural or man-made.[36]

The epidemic-intelligence approach to emerging infections was institutionalized at a global scale over the course of the 1990s as experts from CDC imported the methods of the Epidemic Intelligence Service into WHO. The career of epidemiologist David Heymann is instructive. Heymann began his career in the Epidemic Intelligence Service and in the 1970s worked with CDC on disease outbreak containment in Africa and with WHO on the smallpox eradication program.[37] In the early years of the AIDS pandemic, he helped establish a WHO office that tracked the epidemiology of the disease in developing countries. He then returned to Africa in 1996 to lead the response to a widely publicized Ebola outbreak in Congo, and the director of WHO subsequently asked him to set up a program in emerging diseases. "At this time there was an imbalance in participation internationally in the control of emerging and re-emerging infectious diseases," he later recalled, adding that "the burden was falling mainly on the USA."[38] At WHO, Heymann set up a global funding mechanism that broadened the agency's emerging disease surveillance and response capacities along the CDC model.

As Heymann later remembered, in the wake of the Ebola outbreak, as well as catastrophic outbreaks of cholera in Latin America and plague in India in the early 1990s, a "need was identified" for stronger international coordination of response.[39] A major problem for outbreak investigators was that national governments often did not want to report incidences of diseases that could harm tourism and international trade. The case of the plague outbreak in Surat in 1994, in which Indian officials suppressed international reporting of the event, is often cited as an example of the difficulty of forcing countries to officially acknowledge epidemic outbreaks.[40]

Advocates of the emerging disease problematic suggested revision of the existing International Health Regulations as one potential solution to the problem of national compliance. In the context of emerging diseases, the existing regulations had proved ineffectual in forcing disease notification for two reasons. First, the limited list of reportable conditions—cholera, plague, and yellow fever—was of little relevance for the expansive category of emerging infections; second, there was no way to require countries to actually comply with IHR reporting requirements. As Heymann put it, "in our emerging diseases program our idea was to change the culture so that countries could see the advantage of reporting," but a practical means of enforcing such compliance was needed. The revision of the International Health Regulations became a vehicle by which outbreak investigators could finally construct the functioning global surveillance system that Henderson and others had suggested. Global public health authorities proposed three innovations to the existing regulations that would make it possible for WHO to manage a range of potential disease emergencies.

The first innovation (mentioned above in the context of the Indonesian virus-sharing controversy) responded to the narrow range of conditions to which the existing regulations could be applied. The invention of the concept of the public health emergency of international concern, or PHEIC, vastly expanded the kinds of events to which the regulations might apply. Naturally occurring infectious diseases such as influenza and Ebola, intentional releases of deadly pathogens such as smallpox, or environmental catastrophes such as those that occurred at Bhopal in 1984 and Chernobyl in 1986 could, according to the new regulations, provoke the declaration of a PHEIC. The IHR decision instrument was an important tool for guiding states in determining what would constitute a public health emergency that required the notification of WHO. However, as in the Indonesian H5N1 case, the pathway in the decision instrument defined as "any event of international public health concern" left considerable room for interpretation of the scope of the regulations.

The second major innovation in the revised regulations responded to the concentration of epidemiological knowledge in national public health agencies. The new regulations expanded the potential sources for reports of outbreaks: whereas the previous regulations had restricted actionable reporting to national governments, the revised regulations allowed WHO to recognize reports from nonstate sources such as digital and print media. In this way, a state's unwillingness to report outbreaks would not impede the functioning of the global monitoring system.

The premise was that, given WHO's official recognition of nonstate monitors, media reports of outbreaks could no longer be suppressed by national health officials, and so it would be in a state's interest to allow international investigators into the country as soon as possible in order to undertake disease mitigation measures and assure the public that responsible intervention was under way. The creation during the 1990s of Internet-based reporting systems, such as ProMED in the United States and GPHIN in Canada, that scoured international media for stories about possible outbreaks was critical: with the introduction of these systems, global public health surveillance no longer relied exclusively on state-based epidemiological methods such as the official case report.[41] In 1997, WHO established the Global Outbreak Alert and Response Network (GOARN), a system linking individual surveillance and response networks. The potential for the rapid circulation of infectious disease information undermined national governments' traditional control of public health knowledge, making a global form of disease surveillance possible.

The third major innovation in the revised regulations addressed countries' ability to manage disease outbreaks within their borders. It required that governments build a national capacity for infectious disease surveillance and response. The construction of these national public health institutes on the model of CDC would make possible a distributed global network that relied on the functioning of nodes in each country. Here again, it is worth noting the contrast with the developmentalist model of public health infrastructure. The revised International Health Regulations' reliance on national health systems did not necessarily imply strengthening governmental capacity to manage existing diseases; rather, it sought to direct the development of outbreak detection systems according to the needs of global disease surveillance. As one document put it: "It is proposed that the revised IHR define the capacities that a national disease surveillance system will require in order for such emergencies to be detected, evaluated and responded to in a timely manner."[42] WHO gave countries until 2016 to fulfill this obligation; however, it was unclear where poor countries that already had trouble managing the most common diseases would find the resources for implementing systems for detecting rare or not-yet-existent ones.

Rolling Out the System: SARS

While the revised International Health Regulations were not officially approved by the World Health Assembly until 2005, the SARS outbreak of early 2003 gave Heymann and his colleagues in WHO's emerging diseases division an early opportunity to roll out elements of the agency's new global surveillance and response system. As an outbreak of an unknown and unexpected, but potentially catastrophic viral disease, SARS fit well into the existing category of emerging infectious disease.[43] The Chinese government's initial reluctance to fully report the outbreak led WHO to rely on its new capacity to use nonstate sources of information: the SARS outbreak was the first time the GOARN network identified and publicized a rapidly spreading epidemic. Unlike recalcitrant governments, Heymann said, international scientists "are really willing to share information for the better public good."[44] GOARN made it possible to electronically link leading laboratory scientists, clinicians, and epidemiologists around the world in a virtual network that rapidly generated and circulated knowledge about SARS. WHO closely tracked the spread of the illness and issued a series of recommendations on international travel restrictions. According to Heymann, who led the WHO response, this rapid reaction was key to the containment of the epidemic by July 2003, although he also acknowledged the good fortune of SARS turning out not to be easily transmissible.[45]

The lesson Heymann drew from SARS was that, in a closely interconnected and interdependent world, "inadequate surveillance and response capacity in a single country can endanger the public health security of national populations and in the rest of the world."[46] This was the broad premise underlying global health security as a way of envisioning and managing contagious disease. Processes of globalization—including migration, ecological transformations, and massive international travel—had led to new disease threats that transcended national borders and therefore could not be ignored by wealthy countries. Only a global system of rapidly shared epidemiological information could provide adequate warning in order to mitigate such risks. National sovereignty must accede to the demands of global health security. This lesson was then applied to the next potential disease emergency, avian influenza. As Holbrooke and Garrett argued in calling for Indonesia to comply with WHO's influenza virus–sharing network, SARS had proved that "globally shared health risk demands absolute global transparency."

Applying the New Regulations: XDR-TB

The first invocation of the revised International Health Regulations came in an unexpected context: not the outbreak of a deadly new pathogen in a country in the developing world but the diagnosis of a dangerous strain of tuberculosis in an American air traveler.[47] In the spring of 2007, Atlanta lawyer Andrew Speaker was diagnosed with multidrug-resistant tuberculosis just before leaving for Europe on his honeymoon. Speaker ignored the CDC recommendation not to travel and flew to Europe with his wife. The CDC then informed him by phone that a follow-up test had indicated that he had extensively drug-resistant tuberculosis (XDR-TB), a rare form of the disease that is very difficult to treat. The CDC told Speaker that he would have to either stay in Europe, quarantined in an Italian hospital, or pay his own way back to the United States on a private, medically secure jet. Instead, Speaker bought a commercial plane ticket to Montreal on the Internet and was able to drive into the United States across the Canadian border, even though he had been placed on a Department of Homeland Security watch list. The event briefly caused an international panic, as health officials worried that Speaker had exposed fellow passengers to the pathogen during the long trans-Atlantic flight.

From the vantage of global health security, the Speaker case was a test of the new health preparedness system. As a *New York Times* reporter wrote, "the bizarre case calls into question preparations to deal with medical crises like influenza pandemics and even bioterror attacks."[48] Similarly, a *Los Angeles Times* editorial warned, "One day, a plane landing at LAX could carry a passenger infected with XXDR, a bioterror agent, Ebola or an emerging virus. Will we be ready?"[49] The U.S. House of Representatives' Committee on Homeland Security issued a report on the Speaker incident that linked XDR-TB to the broad problematic of emerging infectious disease. According to the report, addressing this threat would require the integration of public health and security:

> The twin specters of diseases that are increasingly resistant or completely without current treatments and antimicrobials, and the ability of diseases to spread

more quickly than ever before due to rapid transit and other enablers, place public health concerns squarely on the homeland, national, and transnational security agendas. How we address these gaps now will serve as a direct predictor of how well we will handle future events, especially those involving emerging, reemerging, and pandemic infectious disease.[50]

But the Speaker case is far from representative of the global problem of drug-resistant tuberculosis. In fact, the disease is one of the central objects of attention for humanitarian biomedicine.[51] For advocates of humanitarian biomedicine, the case was useful insofar as it drew attention to an underreported issue: the increasing incidence of multidrug-resistant and extensively drug-resistant tuberculosis in parts of the world with poorly functioning public health systems, such as South Africa and the former Soviet Union. As one humanitarian activist urged: "We need to wake up and pay attention to what's happening with TB in other parts of the world. We need to start treating XDR-TB where it is, not just respond to one case of one American who will get the finest treatment."[52] For humanitarian biomedicine, in contrast to global health security, the growing epidemic of drug-resistant tuberculosis pointed to the failures of public health systems to adequately manage a treatable, existing condition among the world's poor.[53]

If the specter of an airplane passenger with XDR-TB was seen as a practice run for a future bioterrorist attack, the questions—and answers—generated by the incident were quite different than if the passenger were seen as a sign of an already existing health emergency, but one taking place outside of the networks and nodes of our own health and communications systems. Thus, the same disease could look quite different, and provoke quite different responses, depending on whether it was taken up within a framework of global health security or one of humanitarian biomedicine.

Conclusion

Whether the revised International Health Regulations would live up to its billing as a radical transformation of international public health intended to provide security against novel pathogens would depend at least in part on its capacity to force sovereign states to comply with

62

the requirements of global health surveillance. The issue of intellectual property rights in the case of Indonesian flu viruses indicates that an alternative way of seeing the problem of global health—one focused on the problem of access to essential medicines in treating existing diseases—could well complicate such efforts. Global health security did not address the major infectious disease problems of the developing world, which were linked to poverty and the lack of resources that could be devoted to basic health infrastructure. As Fidler put it, "the strategy of global health security is essentially a defensive, reactive strategy because it seeks to ensure that States are prepared to detect and respond to public health threats and emergencies of international concern. . . . The new IHR are rules for global triage rather than global disease prevention."[54]

The program of global health security was limited; for example, it did not have any means of addressing the HIV/AIDS pandemic and so did not attract the interest of global health advocates focused on the existing health crisis. It contained no provisions regarding medication access, prevention programs, or research and development for neglected diseases.[55] As critic Philip Calain wrote, describing WHO-led projects such as GOARN, "There is no escaping from the conclusion that the harvest of outbreak intelligence overseas is essentially geared to benefit wealthy nations."[56] Humanitarian biomedicine thus offered potential resources for the critique of what was left out of global health security.

Epilogue: H1N1

Beginning in 2005, the threat of a virulent, easily transmissible strain of H5N1 led to an array of pandemic preparedness measures, including contractual arrangements between national governments and pharmaceutical companies to secure potentially scarce stocks of antiviral medication and flu vaccine in the event of a pandemic. In spring 2009, this preparedness system was put to the test, but in a surprising way: a different subtype of influenza, H1N1, appeared in North America and began to spread to other sites of disease surveillance. Following the International Health Regulations, the spread of H1N1 was named a "public health emergency of international concern" on April 25, and soon after, on June 11, WHO declared a phase 6 pandemic as the virus spread globally. With this declaration, national and international public health agencies were officially put on an emergency footing, and national pandemic preparedness plans were put into action. At this point, it was not that there were already vast numbers of casualties from H1N1 but rather that one could envision a scenario in which such casualties would occur. The task of health officials was to forestall the unfolding of that scenario.

In 2009, European and North American governments spent billions of dollars on procuring H1N1 vaccine and implementing mass immunization campaigns in anticipation of the fall flu season. There was little effort to ensure that vaccine would be available in poor countries. "It's another example of the gap between the north and south," said Michel Kazatchkine, executive director of the Global Fund to Fight AIDS, Tuberculosis and Malaria, as flu season approached. "In the north, vaccines are being stockpiled, antiviral drugs are being stockpiled, all with the risk that these things will not be effective. In the south, there are neither diagnostics nor treatment."[57]

Early the following year, however, the critique of pandemic preparedness measures took a different turn. During the spring of 2010, in Europe and North America, the appropriateness of the intensive public health preparedness efforts that had been undertaken in anticipation of H1N1 began to come under scrutiny. The United States had spent $1.6 billion on 229 million doses of vaccine in what the *Washington Post* called "the most ambitious immunization campaign in U.S. history" but had used less than half the vaccine it had ordered.[58] European countries had for the most part used far less of their available vaccine stocks.

Marc Gentilini, the former president of the French Red Cross, criticized the French government for its "extravagant" spending on the H1N1 vaccination campaign. While France had spent hundreds of millions of euros on H1N1 vaccine purchases from major pharmaceutical companies, less than 10 percent of its population had been vaccinated as of January 2010, and the country sought to unload its excess vaccine supplies. "Preparing for the worst wasn't necessarily preparing correctly," said Gentilini.[59] In turn, President Nicolas Sarkozy defended himself against accusations that the French government had overreacted badly to the threat of pandemic H1N1. "I will always prefer to be too prudent when it comes to people's health than not enough."[60]

Critics argued that billions of dollars spent on vaccines had been squandered in trying to manage a disease that turned out to be less dangerous than seasonal flu. In testimony before the Health Committee of the Council of Europe, German epidemiologist Ulrich Keil accused health agencies of misallocating resources that could have been devoted to diseases that currently kill millions per year: "Governments and public health services are paying only lip service to the prevention of these great killers and are instead wasting huge amounts of money by investing in pandemic scenarios whose evidence base is weak." Others suggested that collective hysteria, or a dark capitalist conspiracy, rather than actual evidence of risk had led to the intensive global response to H1N1. The chair of the Health Committee of the Council of Europe, Wolfgang Wodarg, argued that the pandemic declaration and response was "one of the greatest medical scandals of the century," decrying pharmaceutical industry influence on public health decision making and a "conflict of interest" within the World Health Organization. In June 2010, the *British Medical Journal* reported on the results of the Council of Europe's inquiry: "It pointed to distortion of priorities of public health services, a waste of huge sums of public money, provocation of unjustified fear, and the creation of health risks through vaccines and medications which might not have been sufficiently tested before being authorised in fast-track procedures."[61]

However, the claim that the pandemic declaration—and the billions of dollars of spending on vaccine that followed—resulted from a conflict of interest among WHO experts failed to see the internal logic of WHO's response to H1N1. Once the H1N1 pandemic proved mild, officials were open to accusations that they had acted irrationally at best. However, if one considers the intensive preparedness plans that had been put in place in anticipation of a rapidly spreading, highly virulent form of influenza with the potential to kill millions of people, the question was not whether one would act more or less rationally but which *form of rationality* would determine one's actions. The development, over the preceding two decades, of a system of global health security oriented toward massive intervention *in advance of* a disease catastrophe had made the decision to enact emergency measures at the first signs of potential disaster not just thinkable but, arguably, inevitable.

NOTES

1 The director of WHO's communicable diseases cluster, David Heymann, described GISN as a network that "identifies and tracks antigenic drift and shifts of influenza viruses to guide the annual composition of vaccines, and provides an early alert to variants that might signal the start of a pandemic" David Heymann, "The International Response to the Outbreak of SARS in 2003," *Philosophical Transactions of the Royal Society of London B* 359 (2004): 1127.

2 Aubrey Belford, "Indonesia's Bird Flu Warrior Takes on the World," Agence France-Presse, October 12, 2008.

3 Bryan Walsh, "Indonesia's Bird Flu Showdown," *Time*, May 10, 2007.

4 "International Health Regulations: The Challenges Ahead," *Lancet* 369 (May 26, 2007): 1763.

5 Belford, "Indonesia's Bird Flu Warrior."

6 David P. Fidler, "From International Sanitary Conventions to Global Health Security: The New International Health Regulations," *Chinese Journal of International Law* 4, no. 2 (2005): 325.

7 Cited in David P. Fidler, "Influenza Virus Samples, International Law, and Global Health Diplomacy," *Emerging Infectious Diseases* 14, no. 1 (2008): 92.

8 WHO director-general Margaret Chan, quoted in ibid., 91.

9 U.S. delegation to WHO, quoted in ibid., 92.

10 Ibid.

11 Ibid.

12 Belford, "Indonesia's Bird Flu Warrior."

13 Elizabeth Fee and Dorothy Porter, "Public Health, Preventive Medicine and Professionalization: England and America in the Nineteenth Century," in *Medicine in Society: Historical Essays*, ed. Andrew Wear (Cambridge: Cambridge University Press, 1992).

14 As Foucault noted, population security targets "phenomena that are aleatory and unpredictable when taken in themselves or individually, but which, at the collective level, display constants that are easy, or at least possible, to establish." Michel Foucault, *"Society Must Be Defended": Lectures at the Collège de France, 1975–1976* (New York: Pantheon, 2003), 243.

15 Ibid.

16 George Rosen, *A History of Public Health* (Baltimore, Md.: Johns Hopkins University Press, 1993), 185–86. For the French case, see William Coleman, *Death Is a Social Disease: Public Health and Political Economy in Early Industrial France* (Madison: University of Wisconsin Press, 1982).

17 Thus, as Chadwick's famous 1842 inquiry into living conditions among

the working classes argues, "the expenditures necessary to the adoption and maintenance of measures of prevention would ultimately amount to less than the cost of disease now constantly expanded." Cited in Rosen, *History of Public Health*, 187.

18 For example, as Rosen notes, in designing New York City's diphtheria vaccination campaign among schoolchildren in the 1920s, it was "necessary to know the natural history of diphtheria within the community: How many children of different ages had already acquired immunity, how many were well carriers, and what children were highly susceptible?" Ibid., 312.

19 While I am focusing here on two major strands of Cold War international health, there is a complex history of pre–World War II international health efforts ranging from the Rockefeller Foundation to the League of Nations that historians of public health have recently begun to unravel. See, for example, Alison Bashford, "Global Biopolitics and the History of World Health," *History of the Human Sciences* 19, no. 1 (2006): 67–88.

20 The essential medicines movement, linked to this approach, was a precursor to contemporary efforts to ensure access to biomedical interventions.

21 Theodore M. Brown, Marcos Cueto, and Elizabeth Fee, "The World Health Organization and the Transition from 'International' to 'Global' Health," *American Journal of Public Health* 96, no. 1 (2006): 622–72.

22 By the term "humanitarian biomedicine," I do not refer to a single, clearly articulated framework or tightly linked set of institutions; rather, I mean to indicate a congeries of actors and organizations with diverse histories and missions. They are linked by a sense of the urgency of providing care to suffering victims of violence, disease, and political instability.

23 This section of the chapter draws on portions of Stephen J. Collier and Andrew Lakoff, "The Problem of Securing Health," in *Biosecurity Interventions: Global Health and Security in Question*, ed. Stephen J. Collier and Andrew Lakoff (New York: Columbia University Press, 2008).

24 World Health Organization, *The World Health Report 2007: A Safer Future; Global Public Health Security in the 21st Century* (Geneva: WTO, 2007), 1.

25 Charles Rosenberg has contrasted this new form of "civilizational risk" with those that sparked early public health efforts, noting that anxieties about the risk of modern ways of life are here explained not in terms of the city as a pathogenic environment but in terms of evolutionary and global ecological realities. Charles Rosenberg, "Pathologies of Progress: The Idea of Civilization as Risk," *Bulletin of the History of Medicine* 72, no. 4 (1998): 714–30.

26 World Health Organization, *The World Health Report 2007*, 11.

27   Nicholas King has analyzed the rise of the emerging disease framework
      in detail. See Nicholas King, "Security, Disease, Commerce: Ideologies of
      Post-colonial Global Health," *Social Studies of Science* 32, no. 5–6 (2002):
      763–89.

28   Stephen S. Morse, ed., *Emerging Viruses* (New York: Oxford University
      Press, 1993).

29   Warwick Anderson describes this vision as follows: "Evolutionary processes
      operating on a global scale were responsible for the emergence of 'new'
      diseases. As environments changed, as urbanization, deforestation,
      and human mobility increased, so, too, did disease patterns alter, with
      natural selection promoting the proliferation of microbes in new niches"
      (Warwick Anderson, "Natural Histories of Infectious Disease: Ecological
      Vision in Twentieth Century Bioscience," *Osiris* 19 [2004]: 60).

30   Joshua Lederberg, Robert E. Shope, and Stanley C. Oaks, Jr., *Emerging
      Infections: Microbial Threats to Health in the United States* (Washington, D.C.:
      National Academy Press, 1992); Laurie Garrett, *The Coming Plague: Newly
      Emerging Diseases in a World Out of Balance* (New York: Farrar, Straus and
      Giroux, 1994); Richard Preston, *The Cobra Event* (New York: Ballantine,
      1998).

31   D. H. Henderson, "Surveillance Systems and Intergovernmental
      Cooperation," in *Emerging Viruses*, ed. Stephen S. Morse (New York:
      Oxford University Press, 1993), 27.

32   Susan Wright, "Terrorists and Biological Weapons," *Politics and the Life
      Sciences* 25, no. 1 (2006): 57–115.

33   As Susan Wright (ibid.) argues, the very use of the term "weapons of mass
      destruction" to link nuclear weapons to biological weapons was a strategic
      act on the part of biodefense advocates.

34   The EIS was founded in 1951 by Alexander Langmuir. For Henderson's
      recollections, see D. A. Henderson, *Smallpox: The Death of a Disease* (New
      York: Prometheus, 2009).

35   Alexander Langmuir, "The Surveillance of Communicable Diseases of
      National Importance," *New England Journal of Medicine* 268, no. 4 (1963):
      182–83. As Lyle Fearnley has described, Langmuir pioneered a method
      of epidemiological surveillance designed to track each instance of a
      disease within a given territory, one that would serve the needs of both
      public health and biodefense. Lyle Fearnley, "'From Chaos to Controlled
      Disorder': Syndromic Surveillance, Bioweapons, and the Pathological
      Future," *ARC Working Paper* no. 5 (2005), http://anthropos-lab.net/wp/
      publications/2007/08/workingpaperno5.pdf.

36   Stephen Morse summarized the justification for developing such
      a network: "A global capability for recognizing and responding to

unexpected outbreaks of disease, by allowing the early identification and control of disease outbreaks, would simultaneously buttress defenses against both disease and CBTW. This argues for expanding permanent surveillance programs to detect outbreaks of disease" (Stephen Morse, "Epidemiologic Surveillance for Investigating Chemical or Biological Warfare and for Improving Human Health," *Politics and the Life Sciences* 11, no. 1 [Feb. 1992]: 29).

37 Haroon Ashraf, "David Heymann—WHO's Public Health Guru," *Lancet Infectious Diseases* 4, no. 12 (2004): 785–88.

38 Ibid., 787.

39 David L. Heymann, "The International Response to the Outbreak of SARS in 2003," *Philosophical Transactions of the Royal Society of London B* 359 (2004): 1127.

40 See Garrett, *The Coming Plague.*

41 Lorna Weir and Eric Mykhalovskiy, "The Geopolitics of Global Public Health Surveillance in the 21st Century," in *Medicine at the Border: Disease, Globalization, and Security, 1850–Present*, ed. Alison Bashford (New York: Palgrave MacMillan, 2007), 240–63.

42 World Health Organization, *Revision of the International Health Regulations, Progress Report: Weekly Epidemiological Record*, no. 19 (Geneva, May 10, 2002): 159, quoted in Fidler, "From International Sanitary Conventions," 353.

43 Claire Hooker, "Drawing the Lines: Danger and Risk in the Age of SARS," in *Medicine at the Border: Disease, Globalization, and Security, 1850–Present*, ed. Alison Bashford (Hounsmill, Basingstoke, Hampshire, England, and New York: Palgrave Macmillan, 2007).

44 Ashraf, "David Heymann," 787.

45 Heymann, "International Response," 1129.

46 Ibid., 1128.

47 Howard Markel, Lawrence O. Gostin, and David P. Fidler, "Extensively Drug-Resistant Tuberculosis: An Isolation Order, Public Health Powers, and Global Crisis," *JAMA* 298, no. 1 (2007): 83–86.

48 John Schwartz, "Tangle of Conflicting Accounts in TB Patient's Odyssey," *New York Times*, June 2, 2007.

49 *Los Angeles Times*, "TB Terror," June 10, 2007.

50 House Committee on Homeland Security, *The 2007 XDR-TB Incident: A Breakdown at the Intersection of Homeland Security and Public Health*, 110th Cong., 1st sess., 2007, 2.

51 One example is the recent $33 million initiative by the Gates Foundation, in collaboration with the Chinese ministry of health, to develop a quick diagnostic test for drug-resistant tuberculosis. Sandi Doughton, "Gates

69

Foundation Launches 3rd Initiative in China," *Seattle Times*, March 31, 2009.

52   Dr. Mark L. Rosenberg, quoted in John Donnelly, "Specialists Say TB Case a Sign of Things to Come," *Boston Globe*, June 4, 2007.

53   See, for example, Paul Farmer, *Infections and Inequalities: The Modern Plagues* (Berkeley: University of California Press, 2001).

54   Fidler, "From International Sanitary Conventions," 389.

55   Ibid., 391

56   Philippe Calain, "From the Field Side of the Binoculars: A Different View on Global Public Health Surveillance," *Health Policy and Planning* 22, no. 1 (2007): 19.

57   Michel Kazatchkine and Veronique Martinache, "Swine Flu: Rich Nations' Spending Spurs Ethics Row," Agence France-Presse, August 1, 2009.

58   Rob Stein, "Millions of H1N1 Vaccine Doses May Have to Be Discarded," *Washington Post*, April 1, 2010.

59   Anne Chaon, "France Joins Europe Flu Vaccine Sell-Off," Agence France-Presse, January, 3, 2010.

60   Jeanne Whalen and David Guthier-Villars, "European Governments Cancel Vaccine Orders," *Wall Street Journal*, January 13, 2010.

61   Paul Flynn, quoted in Deborah Cohen and Philip Carter, "WHO and the Pandemic Flu 'Conspiracies,'" *British Medical Journal* 340, no. 12 (June 2010): 1274.

THE AESTHETIC EMERGENCY
OF THE AVIAN FLU AFFECT

Geoffrey Whitehall

The hunt for security leads to a worldwide civil war which destroys all civil coexistence. In the new situation — created by the end of the classical form of war between sovereign states — security finds its end in globalization: it implies the idea of a new planetary order which is, in fact, the worst of all disorders. But there is yet another danger. Because they require constant reference to a state of exception, measure of security work towards a growing depoliticization of society.
— GIORGIO AGAMBEN

The recent film *Chicken Little* presents an interesting twist on a classic childhood fable. Disney rewrites the story of a chicken that believed the sky was falling when in fact it was not; only an acorn had fallen. Instead of being a variation on the story about the boy who cried "wolf," Disney's new rendition replaces a false claim with a real claim. In the new film, the sky *is* falling. Instead of being a story about the desensitizing effects of perpetually using fear and hype to motivate people, *Chicken Little* is about the problem of getting people to act on an

unlikely catastrophic scenario (alien invasion). The reversal of a caution-
ary tale into the story of the end days, and the replacement of prudent
tales with those of Armageddon, are exemplary of a troubling trend in
the contemporary geopolitical imaginary. To justify a national or international response, the contemporary trend requires *making* something
an emergency before it has *become* one. The first section of this chapter
argues that the avian flu emergency embodies a preemptive paradox
that develops an aesthetic-affective mode of governance. This mode of
governance engenders obedience and political will by producing strong
emotional responses. The danger of the avian flu, in effect, lurks in the
affect of its representation. The second section explores the character of
this affective governance in light of a troubling development, the critical shift in contemporary sovereignty that occurs in the zone between
a preemptive state of emergency and an actual state of emergency. In
order to match the aesthetic composition of emergencies like the avian
flu, in other words, the character of sovereignty shifts. As such, a general
internationalized state of exception is replacing nationalized states of
exception. The avian flu both illustrates and facilitates the shift from a
mode of sovereignty that is organized around "national life" toward a
mode of sovereignty that organizes itself on the basis of "human life."
The final section argues that the preemptive paradox of the avian flu
embodies a unique transformative political potential. Intervening in the
avian flu's aesthetic composition can contribute to politicizing the real
state of emergency because human life and animal life become expressions of the same sovereign exception. The material aesthetic in which
the majority of the world's populations (human, chicken, or otherwise)
have become affectively domesticated can be politicized because, in the
name of protecting humanity, human life is revealed to be as expendable as poultry life.

The Aesthetics of Emergency and Its Affect

Like other contemporary crises in the contemporary geopolitical imaginary, the avian flu is fascinating in that, in order to justify a national or
international response from the globally mediated situation room, it has
to be made an emergency even before it becomes one. In language that is
familiar to George W. Bush and Tony Blair (and their "first strike" justifi-

cation for the war on Iraq), Klaus Stöhr, coordinator of the Global Influenza Program of the World Health Organization (WHO), states: "One
of the most difficult things to explain to the public after a pandemic
would be why we weren't prepared, because there have been enough
warnings."[1] Any other decision or discussion appears to be irresponsible.
The age has become exemplary of a preemptive state of emergency.

In addition to being a logical problem akin to the question of which
came first, the chicken or the egg, the preemptive state of emergency
involves aesthetic practices that represent a fact and an interpretation.
The distance between a thing and the social language used to describe
it cannot be definitively stabilized. Constituting a threat to representation, this gap destabilizes the prevailing order of self, community,
and world. Securing this gap and smoothing over the aesthetic distance
between a thing and its sign (the nation, national interest, and the people) have become the cornerstone of responsible politics (representative democracy, advocacy, recognition). Specifically, the discipline of
international relations seeks to annul and/or contain this stealthy gap
in the name of securing the self via the state.[2] Peace, in this sense,
becomes the government management of change and the pacification
of calls for global justice.

In order to decide whether the risks concerning the emergence
and spread of the avian flu are warranted, those inspired by traditional
approaches to international relations might survey the *facts*. In the spirit
of empirical approaches to biosecurity, influenza A is best described as
a dynamic virus that is "constantly emerging"[3] because of its ability to
mutate. These mutations involve rapid evolutionary change and recom-
bination of its two main surface proteins, hemagglutinin (HA) and neur-
aminidase (NA).[4] Although rapidly mutating viruses are natural and
harmless to their host wild birds, when a mutation leaps the species bar-
rier (for example, from ducks to chickens), it has made a potentially
dangerous antigenic shift, a process in which two different virus strains
undergo an abrupt genetic change and form a new subtype. The fallout
of a shift like the H5N1 avian flu has been epidemic spread across Asian,
European, and African poultry stocks. Within the current spread, the
avian epidemic has also caused about 324 human deaths since 2003,
mostly in the Indonesian archipelago. It is important to note, finally, that
a pandemic is different from an epidemic. We are currently in the midst

of an epidemic (animal-to-human transmission). A pandemic emerges when H_5N_1 reassorts, or mixes genetic information, with a human flu so that human-to-human transmission becomes possible. With this antigenic shift, a pandemic human influenza is born.

However, none of these facts, in themselves, amount to saying that *this* threat will become a pandemic. Hence, it is a paradox of preemption. The gap (therefore the threat) persists. Nobody really disputes the potential *risk* of the current epidemic, but nobody can guarantee the facticity of a *dangerous* pandemic emergence. To borrow David Campbell's phrase, "Danger is not an objective condition."[5] The next mutation might lead to a deadly pandemic or to a harmless sniffle. It is impossible to know whether it might happen tomorrow, next year, in a decade, or never again.[6] The difference between a representation of risk and an actual danger is a question of political aesthetics. How the story is told matters. The facts of the avian flu, as such, are less interesting than the aesthetic practices involved in representing the avian flu as an emergency that requires immediate global action. The practices are political because representing something as an enemy has a transformative effect on the very order that is to be protected.

In keeping with the desire to understand the implications of the political aesthetics used to represent an event as an emergency before it has become an emergency, it is useful to explore the practices of representation, or what Dan Smith introduces as "aesthetic comprehension."[7] The term "aesthetic comprehension" is drawn from Gilles Deleuze's engagement with the paintings of Francis Bacon and Immanuel Kant's philosophical exploration of "the role of the imagination (when it is) freed from the legislation of the understanding."[8] Specifically, Bacon's attention to aesthetic comprehension restages the problem of deciding what should count as a sensible part or measure when attempting to understand an event, thing, or composition. The phrase evokes a "lived evaluation"[9] that resides in all practices of understanding. This is slightly different from the important assertion that Roland Bleiker makes in relation to the fall of the World Trade Center's Twin Towers, namely, that when faced with a sublime event, artistic creativity fills the void of understanding.[10] Instead, in order to understand any event (not just sublime ones), aesthetic practices are always already involved in processes of practical and pure understanding.[11] Again, they are involved because the gap between a thing and its sign can never be closed; there is a little sublime in everything.

The textures, tensions, frames, contexts, amplitudes, and durations of a representation also contribute to the affective experience of an event. An affective experience is generally understood to be synonymous with an emotional response. Fear, sadness, and happiness are all affects. However, an attention to affect also emphasizes the somatic intensity that surrounds an emotion.[12] Whereas emotion is a subjective experience, affect $\quad$ **75** is something that is not localized within an individual.[13] Affect might be experienced through the tissues of the mind-body, but it also embodies collective constellations of competing intensities. Panic is as much an individual experience as it is a collective expression of an intense event. A state of becoming panicked can transform into a habit and, sooner or later, become an affective ontology (i.e., a good, vigilant and responsible citizen). Manipulating affective intensities by framing certain stories or magnifying particular images can constitute a kind of affective governance (for example, outrage, tolerance, or melancholy). As Brian Massumi explains, "To treat the emotion as separable . . . from the activation event from which it affectively sprang is to place it on the level of representation. . . . It makes it seem comfortably controllable."[14] Affective governance, therefore, is not only the production of fear in order to *justify* control; it is fear itself. Fear is part of affective governance in a preemptive state of emergency.

Understanding the avian flu's affect involves an aesthetic evaluation of the framings and magnitudes of representation. Take as an example the claim that the H5N1 flu has an apocalyptic kill rate (figures range from 52 percent to 70 percent). The figure's magnitude justifies emergency measures because it contains enough tension and texture to cause serious trepidation. However, these rates are composed from "reported" cases and highlight only patients who were sick enough to require hospital visits. In the words of the American conservative Michael Fumento, "We know the numerator, but without the denominator [these figures are] useless."[15] The actual number of those who become infected remains unknowable. Nevertheless, the tension resonates because it is set within a narrow ribbon of reported cases. It is a sensible part of the constituted distribution. Regardless of whether truthfulness in statistics is ever achievable, the more salient point is that *how* you frame the story about the avian flu matters. In particular, the temporal and spatial aesthetics of representation constitute an affective governance of fear that legitimizes emergency action.

In order to justify calling the avian flu an emergency, temporal representations substitute a future unknown (what if it does happen?) with an immediate unknowable (will it happen?). The chief of microbiology at Mount Sinai Hospital in Toronto, Dr. Donald Low, for example, repeated the aesthetic refrain "the question is not *if* it's going to happen, but *when*."[16] In this spirit, news reports are provocatively titled "The Next Pandemic?"[17] or "The Race against Time."[18] This *waiting* is not an absence of action. Waiting is an all-encompassing action. The anxiety of waiting builds a governmentally useful vigilance in public health.

Drawing from the most extreme historical examples also lubricates the temporal substitution of the plausible "when" for the uncertain "if" and replaces political judgment with an anxious waiting. The avian flu's temporal representation is organized around the 1918 Spanish flu pandemic that killed 20 million to 100 million people around the world because of the conditions created by the brutality of World War I,[19] but it elides the fact that the ominous threshold between epidemic bird flu and pandemic human flu was crossed in 2004.[20] The incident occurred when Pranee Thongchan died from the avian flu virus that she caught from her daughter in Thailand.[21] Although the individual event was tragic for their family and community, these shifts regularly happen without resulting in Armageddon. Nevertheless, the repeated reference to the 1918 Spanish flu makes an aesthetic link that heightens the impending sense of doom. The aesthetic link between 1918 and today occurs either through analogy (the H5N1 flu has the same properties as the 1918 variety) or through refrain (pandemics are cyclical, so we are "overdue").

The aesthetic effect of analogizing between contemporary and historical events results in some catastrophic scenarios. At one extreme, some argue that humanity could be facing numbers like those that Reuters has reported (150 million dead people) or those that Michael Osterholm, director of the Center for Infectious Disease Research and Policy and associate director of the Department of Homeland Security's National Center for Food Protection and Defense, projects (180 million to 360 million dead).[22] Irwin Redlener, director of the national Center for Disaster Preparedness, topped everyone by projecting 1 billion deaths.[23]

At the other extreme, the World Health Organization estimates that the avian flu pandemic is likely to cause between 2 million and 7.4 million deaths globally.[24] The huge difference between 1 billion and 2 million is due to extrapolating from the mild pandemic of 1967, which killed 1 million, or instead the deadly pandemic of 1918.

However, both the aesthetic analogy between 2006 and 1918 and the cyclical refrain about an overdue pandemic, minimize doubts that *this* virus will ever become pandemic. These doubts are justified, for instance, because the analogy between 1918, 1957, 1968, 1997, and 2003 is based, not on a cyclical phenomenon, but on a random set of events.[25] Only unpredictable "cycles" happen in increments of thirty-nine, eleven, twenty-nine, and six years. Therefore elaborate preparation for a random event is not "responsible"; rather, it is hype. The analogous and cyclical aesthetics of the avian flu emergency are a mode of political representation that generates a (de)mobilizing fear.

Although temporality provides the political anticipation and magnitude of the emergency, the spatial aesthetic adds the texture, character, and frame. The daily reporting of virus detection is as much a spatial mapping of an immanent disaster as it is a countdown to doomsday. The updates map a geopolitical trajectory from "here" to "there" and back again. Today, country X,[26] yesterday Nigeria, the day before Turkey and Russia, and everything before that (Cambodia, Vietnam, Thailand, Hong Kong) is the so-called Asian source. From this Asian source, its cousins are stalking Western civilization and getting closer.[27] In Cold War geopolitical form, the West again faces a sentiment popularized by titles such as "The Coming Plague"[28] and "The Coming Anarchy."[29] Instead of the global other being Communism, Africa, and/or Islam, Asia has become (to use the title of Mike Davis's alarming book) "The Monster at *Our* Door."[30]

The spatial framing is crucial to intensifying fear, since hype is about risks being at *our* door. If the risks were at *their* door, to paraphrase the chilling line from the film *Hotel Rwanda*, people would go back to eating their TV dinners.[31]And for the most part, people do. The spatial frame gives the crisis to be faced its political character; it is urgent not only because of its magnitude but also because of its geography. In other words, it becomes important only because it *could* infect us *here*.

Similarly, locating the source in Asia, for instance, puts a specific face on the problem and situates the solution within a geopolitical discourse that seeks to contain the enemy over "there." The critique of spatial frames such as those presented in "The Coming Anarchy" remains compelling. As Simon Dalby argues, the "danger of the [threat] from there compromising the safety of 'here' . . . never countenances the possibility that the economic affluence 'here' is related to the poverty of 'there.'"[32] These encroaching representations, Jorge Fernandez argues, signal a deep anxiety in the Western geopolitical imagination. The fear is that "accelerating cultural and political encounters . . . threaten the nation-state's political viability by heightening the likelihood of conflicts."[33] The imagined cosmopolitan geography is thus at risk.

Furthermore, underlying statements made about the source of the avian flu—cohabitation with chickens, consumption of wild birds—is a geopolitical racism that vilifies other cultures through the aesthetics of hygiene and civilized stratifications (public and private, human and animal).[34] In other words, where threats are localized within *their* cultural practices (instead of *our* international political economies of modern agribusiness), global poverty and environmental destruction become urgent only when they threaten *our* cities, *our* economies, and *our* standards of living.

Given that in times of emergency, it is not polite to point fingers at the root causes of discrimination or exploitation, the avian flu's local contexts have been repackaged by national and international organizations as a universal global threat. The Asian Pacific Economic Cooperation (APEC), for example, elides the specificity of particular challenges (poverty, tuberculosis, tsunamis, or International Monetary Fund policies) and instead expands the flu's spatial ecumene through a universal warning of global economic disaster. In the 2005 APEC meeting Avian and Pandemic Influenza Preparedness and Response, for example, Karen Becker reported, "There is danger *everywhere*. No economy on Earth can afford to ignore this threat [since] interruption of supply chains could leave *us* without essential goods and products, particularly in this day of just-in-time manufacturing."[35] Through this universal spatial representation, the whole world is back to being the West's lifeboat, and everything that led to the flood is forgotten.

Attending to the aesthetic representation of the avian flu emergency gives a different context to Stöhr's cumulative warnings that "there is no doubt there will be another pandemic"[36] and that "We are living on borrowed time."[37] The danger exists in WHO's representation of the ten key facts that everyone needs to know: (1) pandemic influenza *is* different from avian influenza, (2) influenza pandemics *are* recurring events, (3) the world *may* be on the brink of another pandemic, (4) all countries *will* be affected, (5) widespread illness *will* occur, (6) medical supplies *will* be inadequate, (7) large numbers of deaths *will* occur, (8) economic and social disruption *will* be great, (9) every country *must* be prepared, (10) WHO will alert the world *when* the pandemic threat increases.[38] In this list, the use of definitive verbs ("is," "are," "will," and "must") blends with the singular use of a modal verb ("may be") and justifies WHO's authority to decide the governing protocols for political action ("must," "when"). Beyond the capacity of any one particular state, an imminent danger has been created out of a transcendental "unknown" by rooting an aesthetic emergency in a substantiated affect of fear. Therefore, everyone must become *prepared* for when, where, and how WHO decides it is necessary to act.

State decision makers and international officials have blurred the boundary between a preemptive state of emergency and an actual state of emergency. This blurring requires transforming the way in which decisions are made and how sovereignty functions.

International Relations and the State of Emergency

The proliferating attention to the term "state of emergency" could be embraced as a confirmation of Walter Benjamin's eighth thesis on history: "The tradition of the oppressed teaches us that the 'state of emergency' in which we live is not the exception but the rule."[39] History is replete with examples that support this thesis.[40] A state of emergency comprises the proliferating interpretive aesthetic-affective frameworks that normalize human and environmental life. How the avian flu emergency is politically reproduced reveals the degree to which a state of emergency has become a rule of everyday life.

This is not the same thing as saying that the reproduction of a state of emergency coincides with the numerical frequency of events that necessitate emergency powers (Hurricanes Katrina and Rita, the Indonesian tsunami, September 11), nor does it reflect what has been called a "culture of fear" in the media.[41] Instead, something more interesting is occurring. The state of emergency is the actualization of a particular view of international relations and U.S. foreign policy that defines peace as the constant preparation for war. Giorgio Agamben explains as follows:

President Bush's decision to refer to himself constantly as the "Commander in Chief of the Army" after September 11, 2001, must be considered in the context of this presidential claim to sovereign powers in emergency situations. If, as we have seen, the assumption of this title entails a direct reference to the state of exception, then Bush is attempting to *produce a situation* in which the emergency becomes the rule and the very distinction between peace and war (and between foreign and civil war) becomes impossible.[12]

Instead of saying that George Bush's politics lead to contemporary fascism in the United States,[43] a more politically important point needs to be developed. What is interesting in the U.S example is that, from wiretapping U.S. citizens and suspending habeas corpus to subjecting enemy combatants to extraordinary rendition, and from Iraq to Kosovo and back to Iraq again, U.S. security discourse is embodying a *shift* from national juridical law to international exceptional politics. A nationalized state of emergency has made *an antigenic shift*—to borrow the epidemiological term—to an internationalized state of emergency. This shift pivots around the concept of sovereignty.

Sovereignty is both an epistemological and an ontological event. It is a way of becoming organized in the world. In an epistemological sense, sovereignty becomes the means through which some statements come to have legitimacy (for example, "rational," "fact," or "progressive") while others are negated (for example, "emotion," "opinion," and "tradition"). These decisions simultaneously constitute a series of ontological friend/enemy distinctions,[44] oppositions that are constitutive of both the nationalized subject who creates and the nation of subjects who are created.[45] In this sense, sovereignty unfolds "by exercising (the) right to kill, or by refraining from killing."[46] It also includes the more contemporary manifestation of simply "letting die."[47] Sovereignty is simultaneously the decision between who lives and who dies and the qualification of a life worth living. The political problem of sovereignty, therefore, does not lie with *proper* categorization of this life versus that other life. Instead, the political regime of sovereignty functions in the very act of *categorizing* life.

As such, sovereignty makes a declaration of emergency possible through the act of categorization itself. To modify Carl Schmitt's definition in an important way, sovereignty is *how* the exception is made.[48] It is how a risk becomes a danger, an inside becomes an outside, and a state of peace becomes a state of emergency. Drawing a staunch line between friend and enemy, for example, evokes an aesthetic practice of metaphysical conceit. This conceit, or founding violence, has become normalized as state sovereignty and as a nationalized state of exception.

Returning to the earlier point, an antigenic shift has occurred between the nationalized state of exception and the internationalized state of exception that organizes around the proliferation of global emergencies like the avian flu. Michel Foucault identified an "earlier" shift between a classic and disciplinary mode of sovereignty in which "wars are no longer waged in the name of a sovereign who must be defended; they are waged on behalf of the existence (national life) of everyone; entire populations are mobilized for the purpose of wholesale slaughter in the name of life necessity: massacres have become vital."[49] Another shift is occurring today. Instead of protecting life in national terms (defending citizens), an internationalized state of exception is organized around the protection of humanity.[50] An internationalized clamor of global friend/ enemy decisions and normal/abnormal classifications is thus materializing. Whereas a nationalized state of exception materializes through an aesthetic-affective framework of international emergencies, an internationalizing state of exception is materializing through the proliferation of global emergencies (avian flu, terrorism, financial crises).

The pressing question, however, becomes what forms of sovereignty emerge when wars are fought and emergencies contained, not for a national biological population, but for humanity's biological survival and for human life itself? How is the line drawn in this context? What type of line can be drawn in this context? When categorization loses its sovereign function, the result is a shift to preemption, responsibility to protect, and the precautionary principle. If this proposition holds, then the line between friend and enemy is no longer drawn spatially; the line has become a temporal function. Preemptive governance, as such, is the governing of the present from the standpoint of a presumed future. It pivots on the disappearance of the nationalized individual and the biopolitical emergence of a different ontological face.[51]

Anne Caldwell argues that humanitarian intervention represents a new form of global power called "bio-sovereignty." Her argument pushes beyond Schmitt's hesitancy about creating a political category called "humanity." Schmitt had argued that the category "humanity" would negate the defining moment of politics (that is, deciding who is friend and who is enemy).[52] For Caldwell, however, "[a]t least since the end of the cold war, humanity has emerged as a material political group in the same manner that 'the people' became a concrete group with the rise of the representative nation-state. . . . What political power represents humanity is less apparent."[53] In other words, new preemptive humanitarian actions constitute the nascent normalization of an international state of exception. Caldwell states: "The impossibility of locating sovereignty in a precise territory or group does not signal a collapse of sovereignty, but its transformation."[54] As such, the United Nations and World Health Organization do not check sovereign power; they open up avenues for sovereign transformation, redemption, and rejuvenation.

This sovereign transformation, or, rather, transformation of sovereignty, proceeds in, through, and upon the new materializing body called "humanity." Reflecting on Giorgio Agamben's work, Caldwell argues that "[h]umanity, rather than serving as a limit on sovereignty, appears as its medium and product." In other words, Caldwell explains, "[a]s sovereignty expands beyond the nation state form, it increasingly operates as bio-sovereignty: a form of sovereignty operating according to the logic of exception rather than law, applied to material life rather than juridical life, and moving within a global terrain now almost exclusively bio-political."[55] Pushing Caldwell's definition further, bio-sovereignty preemptively decides between life and a life unworthy of life in a radically decentralized and highly mobile set of decisions, technologies, networks and affective constellations.

As such, new preemptive global practices of sovereignty are emerging and becoming recognizable in the name of protecting humanity from the next pandemic. In his opening statement to the APEC Health Task Force, an initiative born out of an earlier SARS scare, Amar Bhat suggests that the "human and economic cost of an uncontained influenza pandemic could be horrifying. We have a humanitarian obligation (as officials and individuals) . . . to do our part."[56] Bhat's plea appears innocent; however, we do not know what "doing our part" entails. Who lives, who dies, and who decides, and how, why, and when?

In the midst of an international state of emergency, a new "Global Triage" constitutes its own necessity; a centralizing and decentralizing sovereignty becomes an "objective condition."[57] Ceremonially citing the "lack of international harmony,"[58] a permanent global task force becomes necessary in order to deal with the next pandemic. Such a force would include international agencies such as the World Health Organization, the Food and Agriculture Organization of the United Nations, and the World Organisation for Animal Health. The task force would need to seamlessly integrate U.S. organizations such as the Department of Health and Human Services, Centers for Disease Control and Prevention, National Institutes of Health, and the Food and Drug Administration. It would also need to incorporate the European equivalents. Other regional organizations, including, in Asia, APEC, the Association of Southeast Asian Nations, the Asian Resource Foundation, and the Asian Development Bank, could not be omitted, nor could European or even African organizations. Local authorities and multinational pharmaceutical companies must also be asked to cooperate. A governmental nexus himself, Michael Osterholm, director of the Center for Infectious Disease Research and Policy and associate director of the National Center for Food Protection and Defense, declared that "[p]andemic planning must be on the agenda of every school board, manufacturing plant, investment firm, mortuary, state legislature and food distributor (in the world)."[59] The scope and scale of planning is simply awesome.

What we are witnessing is not a unified global government; instead, this global triage amounts to empowering a monotony of people to make (seemingly) mundane choices about the vital characteristics of life.[60] The APEC Health Task Force, for example, convenes to discuss regional and global responses to the avian flu threat and claims to do nothing more extraordinary than having its members "simply share information, lessons, and advice to help facilitate more efficient and effective responses."[61] A typical call to *global action* includes nothing more exciting than the following claim:

Specific monitoring of virological, serological and clinical parameters is urgently needed for people at risk. Also needed are detailed autopsies to characterize the disease, and the subsequent establishment of appropriate animal models to evaluate available intervention strategies. For poultry, bird populations should be actively surveyed for all types of flu viruses, using high-throughput technology; production and distribution systems should be modified; and stricter adherence to contamination measures achieved when there is an outbreak.[62]

However mundane these choices might sound, they will amount to extraordinary circumstances for someone somewhere.

The implications from this global triage are most obvious in the relations between humans, viruses, and birds. In this threat scenario, bird and viruses will be exterminated in order to save humans. The decisions become more difficult, however, when choosing among human lives. Laurie Garrett has warned that only about 500 million people could be vaccinated, about 14 percent of the world's population. On April 1, 2005, President Bush issued an "executive order authorizing the use of quarantines inside the United States and permitting the isolation of international visitors . . . [i]f one country implements such orders, others will follow suit."[63] This is no prank. Given the U.S. precedent of not sharing vaccines, established during the 1976 H1N1 crisis, it is unlikely that *all* humanity will be saved. To the degree that global biological apartheid does not already exist as the de jure norm of international relations, there is simply not enough Tamiflu to go around. The global triage will decide how, when, and where to create quarantines, cull populations, establish no-travel zones, and distribute antiviral drugs.[64] If the occasion arises, how will the decision between life and death be made?

Once again, in the name of humanity, the affluent will likely be saved from the fate imposed on the rest. In order to meet the needs of the rest, the Ontario Health Plan for an Influenza Pandemic convened a working group of clinicians with expertise in critical care, infectious diseases, medical ethics, military medicine, triage, and disaster management with the task of creating a critical care triage protocol.[65] Deciding who lives and dies in the emergency will depend on a sequential organ failure assessment score. The triage has "4 main components: inclusion criteria, exclusion criteria, minimum qualifications for survival and a prioritization tool."[66] Life-and-death decisions rest in other people's hands. Backed by a set of guidelines, they will prescribe courses of action as if their propositions were not in themselves ethically, politically, and emotionally contentious.

However, conversations about life and death are much more complicated when the illusion of modern sovereignty slips from the hands of a single individual (the president or the doctor). Aihwa Ong and Steven Collier call these new ways of deciding, new moments of decision, and new kinds of governance "global assemblages."[67] These global assemblages are constituted by a series of overlapping calls of emergency, demands for preemptive action, and a contemporary episteme that slowly claims the name of humanity. The result is a new population, a new essence of humanity, and a new appreciation of life, called "biovalue."[68] Biology establishes citizenship, rights, and responsibilities. According to this means of valuation, explains Nikolas Rose, biological citizenships "encompass all those citizenship projects that have linked their concepts of citizens to beliefs about the biological existence of human beings, as individuals, as families and lineages, as communities, as population and race and as a species."[69] These linkages occur well before an emergency has begun through a medicalization and pharmaceuticalization of life (with initiatives such as the human genome project, stem-cell research, AIDS research, and organ harvesting).[70] A biological and technological indistinction emerges in the encoding, recoding, and decoding of contemporary biomedical research.[71] Eugene Thacker calls this the "optimization of biology."[72] Signaling a radical transformation and dislocation of thinking about the future of human life, biological citizenship and biomedical research protect and optimize life by simultaneously minimizing what it can mean.

As the indistinction between forms of biological life becomes possible, the conditions for a preemptive global triage emerges. Human life becomes chicken life through sickness, and chicken life becomes viral life through infection. "What would thus be obtained," Agamben explains, "is neither an animal life nor a human life, but only a life that is separated and excluded from itself—only a bare life."[73] What emerges, in fact, is *infected life*. In the narrative of the "next pandemic," the same technologies of control, surveillance, containment, vaccination, and extermination will constitute the indistinction between human, chicken,

H5N1, and antiviral life. Quarantines and dead zones will be shaped around how life is appreciated through a battlefield triage.

The risk of war, as Carl von Clausewitz presented it, rests in the escalating logic that leads toward total war.[74] From *a* war to *the* war to end *all* wars, greater and greater applications of violence are justified in the majesty of the objective—saving humanity. Replacing the nuclear shadow of World War II, the twilight of the next pandemic makes civilian casualties managerially expendable. This risk, however, rests as much with peace as with war. When overlapping appeals to emergency powers govern everyday life, then, as Stöhr warns, "we are living on borrowed time."[75] Most of us (now speaking inclusively of chickens and viruses, too) are already planned casualties, biomedical collateral in the very war to protect human life.[76] As such, the living dead wait in suspended tension between panic and docility, caught between stockpiling Tamiflu and nervously consuming Kentucky Fried Chicken. This global triage in particular and emerging preemptive governance in general are what Benjamin calls the "real" state of emergency that is "the monster at the door."[77]

The Material Aesthetics of Resistance

The monstrosity of an internationalized state of emergency and global triage sounds less menacing when put into the context of the aesthetic-affective governance of the avian flu emergency. The only threat greater than the avian flu emergency, experts warn, is the threat of becoming complacent about an imminent danger. The APEC task force reports that the greatest barriers to influenza preparedness were the ministers' lack of "interest," absence of "funding" and "international collaboration" on surveillance, poor risk communication, and the difficulty of securing vaccine and antiviral supplies.[78] From the standpoint of APEC, when the barriers to creating a global system of societal controls are motivation, funds, and collaboration, then it seems completely "reasonable" to suggest that the remedy is generating the appropriate aesthetic- political will (i.e., panic).

Creating panic amounts to emotional brinkmanship. Any other course of action besides panic appears to be simultaneously irrelevant and suicidal. Emotional brinkmanship eventually becomes the all-encompassing term "preparedness." As if such a response can only be represented through a cinematic montage, ABC released its horrifying TV movie *Fatal Contact: Bird Flu in America* in order to secure the appropriate frenetic mix of hope and despair from the public.[79] The *New York Times*, acknowledging that the use of panic has the potential for replicating Orson Welles's *War of the Worlds* broadcast, warned that its article about preparing "for a real outbreak of avian flu" (part of the article's very title) was "not a real article." It was only an "exercise."[80] In fact, Donald McNeil, Jr., was reporting on the CDC's first "fully functional" simulation of an avian flu emergency. Again, a cinematic aesthetic was employed to represent the news. McNeil reported, "[l]ike an episode of the television program '24' the drill was supposed to be taking place in real time" and therefore resulted in its own "movie-within-the-movie moments." He concluded by recounting the words of Peter Taylor, the man behind the scenes "pulling the strings . . . in a little room upstairs known as the Simulation Cell." When asked if the human race survives, "Taylor gave only a hint: the exercise never really ends," revealing the underlying logic of preemptive governance. When Orson Welles, Jack Bauer, and the Wizard of Oz are all represented in one *New York Times* article, that is certainly enough to reassure everyone that everything will work out fine in the end; that is, if we don't all die first.

Identifying the emergence of this troubling trend, Paul Virilio notes, "No one is waiting anymore for the revolution, only for the accident, the breakdown, that will reduce this unbearable chatter to silence."[81] Facing a bio-nano-tech future and looming social and environmental disasters, proponents of a preemptive state of emergency and its most outspoken critics are ironically united by the slogan of the 1909 Futurist Manifesto, "War is the world's only Hygiene."[82] This paralyzing chatter forces politics into a corner where the only options are to contribute to the state of emergency and/or dream of the total economic and political collapse of the "real" state of emergency.

This political paralysis combines two aspects of Walter Benjamin's project, the first of which is embodied in his lament for the angel of history depicted in Paul Klee's painting *Angelus Novus*.

[A]n angel looking as though he is about to move away from something he
is fixedly contemplating. His eyes are staring, his mouth open, his wings are
spread. This is how one depicts the angel of history. His face is turned toward

the past. Where we perceive a chain of events, he sees one single catastrophe which keeps piling wreckage upon wreckage and hurls it in front of his feet. The angel would like to stay, awaken the dead, and make whole what has been smashed. But a storm is blowing from Paradise; it has got caught in his wings with such violence that the angel can no longer close them. This storm irresistibly propels him into the future to which his back is turned, while the pile of debris before him grows skyward. This storm is what we call progress.[83]

The aesthetic composition of this image is compelling because of the way that the viewer is drawn into the diagram of the painting (the edges are darkened, and it almost looks as if smoke is looming in the background). This tension builds through Klee's childlike bridge between abstraction and realism in the awkward figure of the angel. Perhaps this angel of history's remarkable resemblance to a chicken is inconsequential; however, it allows a further analogy to made about framing. The same modern aesthetic composition blackmails the angel and the alarmists who demand that we act responsibly in the face of the avian flu emergency. Together, the new pandemicists and the angel of history stand staring, mouths open, and arms spread, paralyzed, docile, stupefied, and caged by fear.

The second component of this political paralysis is Benjamin's insistence that we overcome the fate of Klee's "angelic chicken." To this end, Benjamin differentiates between a state of emergency and a *real* state of emergency. The real state of emergency transforms the state of emergency into a political struggle that radically reorganizes the material conditions of modern society.

The tradition of the oppressed teaches us that the "state of emergency" in which we live is not the exception but the rule. We must attain to a conception of history that is in keeping with this insight. Then we shall clearly realize that it is *our task to bring about a real state of emergency, and this will improve our position in the struggle against Fascism*. One reason why Fascism has a chance is that in the name of progress its opponents treat it as a historical norm . . . [84]

Bringing about the real state of emergency is a messianic project of reinvigorating the political. This occurs in two steps. The first is to politicize the historical norm of the state of emergency already under way. The second is to build a material aesthetic resistance sufficient to this development. It is at the juncture of these two political vectors that the political question of aesthetic composition becomes a critical political resource.

The first vector requires reinvigorating the political, which, Agamben argues, "has suffered a lasting eclipse because it has been contained by law."[85] Reinvigorating the political, in this sense, would require re-politicizing the relationship between life and law. Law and its sovereign founding violence would no longer be the constitutive condition for modern life.[86] Instead, politics would occupy the "emptiness"[87] in between law and life and become a space for "human action."[88] Politics would become "a counter movement that, working in an inverse direction in law and in life, always seeks to loosen what has been artificially and violently linked."[89] Subverting the very state of emergency that gives law in general or, in this case, global surveillance its legitimacy and ontological necessity, a creative politics does not attempt to reimpose a normalized sovereign rule of law. Instead, by revealing the political nature of the state of emergency's normalized rule of law, it politicizes the aesthetic-affective boundaries that manage and produce the state of emergency.

Although its development exceeds the scope of this chapter, such a creative politics requires keeping the metaphysical boundaries between human, animal, and viral life open in order to offer the possibility of a new future solidarity.[90] If the avian flu is a form of human governance that requires thinking about other animals as either food, pets, or wild, then politicizing this sovereign exception would engender a "human politics" that would involve developing a different relationship with the animal inside the human and the human inside the animal.[91] Without politically opening the insecurities that constitute humanity, the fate of animals will become the fate of (some?) humans.

The second vector requires affirming political openness while pluralizing the political tactics available. The paralyzing force of the avian flu emergency's affective blackmail operates by making an uncertain future a governable resource. In this formulation, fear of the future does not precede the operability of this uncertainty; fear *is* the affective governance of a preemptive state of emergency. That affective governance, or what Brian Massumi calls "activation," is the production of fear itself.[92] In other words, we are not afraid first; fear is the experience of an operation (political control). Citing William James, Massumi explains: "We don't run because we are afraid, we are afraid because we run." Paralysis sets in because the "emergence of emotion preempts action. Actual action has been short-circuited."[93] Political paralysis becomes a habit, a habit of becoming, in which an affective consensus constitutes the political limits of life itself.

In the middle of an affective buildup, it is unlikely that a calming call to reevaluate the categories used to frame the problem will break the panic habit. The affect is too great. The ABC drama *Fatal Contact: Bird Flu in America*, for example, represents the total reification of fear. In the drama, dead bodies are dumped in parking lots, the death toll spirals out of control, and helpless fathers commit suicide in front of their children. In the face of such a representation, docility seems justified. Perhaps the drama would be harmless if it led only to a spike in sales of canned goods and emergency candles. If it bolsters contemporary justifications for fueling proliferating states of emergency, however, then the aesthetic composition of the pandemic needs to be targeted as a site of political significance.

It is possible to disrupt the aesthetic composition of the avian flu emergency and invite a pluralization of creative political possibilities. This is already under way. For example, the proliferation of political satire is illustrative of a strategy that recontextualizes the aesthetic comprehension of the avian flu pandemic by employing measures other than the 1918 flu pandemic. *Late Show with David Letterman*, the *Colbert Report*, and the *Daily Show with Jon Stewart*, in particular, have opened up a different way of comprehending "unavoidable Armageddon." Their satirical accounts of *Fatal Contact*, for instance, use a different lived evaluation (for example, the Cold War, the killer bees, Y2K, or the war on terror) as an aesthetic measure. Instead of trying to solve the problem of the avian flu, they target the constitutive relationship between emergency law and life and open it to political evaluation.

In other words, with a different aesthetic measure, the nature of the emergency and the form of governance could change. For example, the world community is spending $1.9 billion[94] to confront a potential risk of 2 million to 7 million deaths instead of directing these funds toward the routine pandemic killers of tuberculosis (annually, 8.8 million cases and 2 million dead), malaria (5 billion episodes and more than 1 million deaths a year), or AIDS (2.9 million new infections a year and 25 million in total).[95] Similarly, the U.S. contribution to the global avian flu effort diverts funds from existing emergency and preparedness commitments, such as tsunami relief for Southeast Asia, where the economic and political vulnerability to avian flu is actually greatest.[96] Such examples demonstrate where the line between qualified and unqualified life resides and whom the "international" community cares about most.[97]

When the aesthetic measures shift from mapping migrating birds, human-induced emergencies become a potential cause of future global pandemics, since they (like all aspects of globalization) create the very web of interconnections that avian flu cannot develop on its own. For example, the following chilling event occurred in October 2004:

> The American College of Pathologists mailed a collection of mystery microbes prepared by a private lab to almost 5,000 labs in 18 countries for them to test as part of their recertification. The mailing should have been a routine procedure; instead in March 2005 a Canadian lab discovered that the test included a sample of H2N2 flu—a strain that killed 4 four million people worldwide in 1957. H2N2 has not been in circulation since 1968, meaning that hundreds of millions of people lack immunity from it. Had any of the samples leaked or been exposed to the environment, the results could have been devastating. On learning of the error, the WHO called for the immediate destruction of all the test kits.[98]

Repeatedly, the very problems that stalk humanity are created by humans' attempts to contain the threats they face. The way in which emergencies are produced and managed constitutes the real emergency. There is a failure to recognize that threats are not isolated from the affective governance that created them.

Similarly, the emergency looks different when the threat of bird flu has less to do with birds than it does with the political economy of industrial food production. For instance, an article in *New Scientist* in January 2004 reported that the source of the 2003 H5N1 super-virus that emerged in Hong Kong was "a combination of official cover-up and questionable farming practices."[99] Specifically, Chinese growers had accelerated the evolution of the H5N1 super-strain by immunizing their chickens with an inactivated virus in order to safeguard industrial-scale production.[100] Simply put, if Tyson Foods incarcerates and slaughters 2.2 billion chickens annually, it creates vast amplifiers of viral risks. The expedient way to minimize the avian flu risk, therefore, is not color-coordinating surgical masks and organizing photo opportunities for government officials to eat chicken lunches that *imply* something "real" is being done. Rather, it involves changing the most basic material relationships that constitute the current human picture. Industrial agricultural production needs to be made a political problem if the future of viral infections is to be, not

managed, but renegotiated.

Failing to condemn capitalism's "human-induced environmental shocks" and "corporate livestock revolutions"[101] that are actively championed by the World Bank, the International Monetary Fund, and regional organizations like Asian Pacific Economic Cooperation, the Association of Southeast Asian Nations, and the Asian Development Bank serves only to reproduce a hysterical sense of danger that stands in for political debate. These responses only mask the very practices of impoverishment that champion industrial agriculture and economic specialization while reducing culturally specific and traditionally rooted support networks. Modernity panics because its abstract plans cannot be rooted and rehearsed in local practices based in historical knowledge that create pluralities of well-being.

Conclusion

Instead of reproducing the contemporary theme of Disney's *Chicken Little*, a material aesthetic resistance invokes the political skepticism engendered through Aesop's fable "The Boy Who Cried Wolf." This prudent story ends with the moral of the story that *even when liars tell the truth, nobody believes them.* The beginning of the fable might prove more even more interesting, however. It offers a boy, who is so bored with his own existence, as if it were as dull as a chicken's, that he decides to entertain himself by crying "wolf." This is our condition. In a world in which the human-chicken-virus distinction has already collapsed in the singularity of boredom and fear, the call of emergency becomes not only more likely but apolitical. Perhaps as appreciations of different degrees of fear develop, a wider affirmation of lived risks will replace the pandemic blackmail of fear. When opened politically, the aesthetic emergency loses its affective weight. In turn, it becomes more palatable to call for sustained social, economic, and environmental transformation.

The irony is that the *expedient and responsible* political response to avian flu does not involve empowering a global plutocracy, a global triage, to manage every risk as if it were a world-ending danger. It involves changing the way in which human organization relates to the world in which it is embedded. Simple "conservative" solutions such as empowering local food networks and taking responsibility for socio-ecological footprints will do much more to reduce future threats than utopian solutions such as global surveillance or full-spectrum dominance.[102] This is not to avoid the scale of the avian flu problem. On the contrary, what is required is nothing short of a sustained reorganization of humanity's relationship within its animal and environmental self. What form this aesthetic material affirmation may take, however, is unknowable, because in each instance, resistance writes its own aesthetic and affective geography.[103] This spread of political possibility might also constitute a world that is viable and resistant to future human-made problems, like the avian flu, the global model of industrial food production, or the global triage itself.

NOTES

Epigraph from Giorgio Agamben, "Security and Terror," trans. Carolin Emcke, *Theory & Event* 5, no. 4 (2001).

1   Quoted in Mike Davis, *The Monster at Our Door: The Global Threat of Avian Flu* (New York: The New Press, 2005), 139.

2   Richard Ashley, "Living on the Borderlines: Man, Poststructuralism and War," in *International/Intertextual Relations*, ed. James Der Derian and Michael Shapiro (Lexington, Ky.: Lexington Books, 1989), 259–321.

3   Jeffrey K. Taubenberger and Ann H. Reid, "Archavevirology: Characterization of the 1918 'Spanish' Influenza Pandemic Virus," in *Emerging Pathogens*, ed. Charles Greenblatt and Mark Spigelman (Oxford: Oxford University Press, 2003), 189, quoted in Davis, *The Monster at Our Door*, 11.

4   Davis, *The Monster at Our Door*, 11.

5   David Campbell, *Writing Security: United States Foreign Policy and the Politics of Identity* (Minneapolis: University of Minnesota Press, 1998), 1.

6   See also François Ewald, "Insurance and Risk," in *The Foucault Effect: Studies in Governmentality*, ed. Graham Burchell, Colin Gordon, and Peter Miller (Chicago: University of Chicago Press, 1991), 199.

7   Daniel W. Smith, introduction to *Francis Bacon: The Logic of Sensation*, by Gilles Deleuze (Minneapolis: University of Minnesota Press, 2002), xvii.

8   Ibid.

9   Ibid., xviii.

10 Roland Bleiker, "Art after 9/11," *Alternatives: Global, Local, Political* 31, no. 1 (2006): 80.

11 See Jacques Rancière, *The Politics of Aesthetics: The Distribution of the Sensible* (New York: Continuum, 2004), 12–19.

12 Brian Massumi, *Parables for the Virtual* (Durham, N.C.: Duke University Press, 2002), 27.

13 Ibid.

14 Brian Massumi, "Fear (the Spectrum Said)," *Positions* 12, no. 1 (2005): 39.

15 Michael Fumento, "Fuss and Feathers: Pandemic Panic over the Avian Flu," *Weekly Standard*, November 21, 2005, 28.

16 Quoted in Margot Andresen, "Avian Flu: WHO Prepares for the Worst," *Canadian Medical Journal* 170, no. 4 (March 2004): 777.

17 See Canadian Broadcasting Corporation, "The Next Pandemic?" available at http://www.cbc.ca/news/background/avianflu.

18 Anthony Fauci, "Race against Time," *Nature* 435 (May 26, 2005): 423–24.

19 Davis, *The Monster at Our Door*, 124–25.

20 Dr. Klaus Stöhr, who headed WHO's H5N1 outbreak response, reports that the 1997 Hong Kong strain did mutate into a form that was transmissible between humans, but because of its relative weakness, it caused few illnesses (Andresen, "Avian Flu," 777).

21 Davis, *The Monster at Our Door*, 4–8.

22 Number quoted in Fumento, "Fuss and Feathers," 24.

23 Redlener later clarified that he meant to say 1 billion sick. See ibid.

24 Ibid., 29.

25 Ibid., 30.

26 After debating whether to change this country based on current news reports, I decided to leave it as "country X."

27 For an interactive map showing how the contagion is getting closer, see news.bbc.co.uk/2/shared/spl/hi/world/05/bird_flu_map/html/1.stm.

28 Laurie Garrett, *The Coming Plague: Newly Emerging Diseases in a World Out of Balance* (New York: Farrar, Straus and Giroux, 1994).

29 Robert Kaplan, "The Coming Anarchy," *Atlantic Monthly* 273, no. 2 (1994): 44–76.

30 See Davis, *The Monster at Our Door* (emphasis added).

31 *Hotel Rwanda*, dir. Terry George (MGM, 2004).

32 Simon Dalby, "Reading Kaplan's 'Coming Anarchy,'" in *The Geopolitics Reader*, ed. Gearóid Ó Tuathail, Simon Dalby, and Paul Routledge (London: Routledge, 1998), 199.

33 Jorge Fernandez, "Ebola Takes to the Road," in *Sovereign Lives: Power in Global Politics*, ed. Jenny Edkins, Michael J. Shapiro, and Véronique Pin-Fat (London: Routledge, 2004), 192.

34 Anne McClintock, *Imperial Leather: Race, Gender and Sexuality in the Colonial Conquest* (London: Routledge, 1995), chapters 1 and 5.

35 Karen Becker, "Avian and Influenza Pandemics: A Threat to the Asia-Pacific Community," submitted to APEC Meeting on Avian and Pandemic Influenza Preparedness and Response, Brisbane, Australia 31 October–1 November 2005, available at http://unpan1.un.org/intradoc/groups/public/documents/apcity/unpan022560.pdf (emphasis added)

36 "WHO Warns of Dire Flu Pandemic," CNN, available at http://www.cnn.com/2004/Health/11/25/birdflu.warning/.

37 Klaus Stöhr, quoted in Davis, *The Monster at Our Door*, 165.

38 World Health Organization, "Ten Concerns If Avian Influenza Becomes a Pandemic," World Health Organization, http://www.who.int/csr/disease/influenza/pandemic10things/en/ (emphasis added).

39 Walter Benjamin, "Thesis on the Philosophy of History," in *Illuminations: Essays and Reflections*, ed. Hannah Arendt (New York: Schocken Books, 1968), 257.

40 See Mark Neocleous, "The Problem with Normality: Taking Exception to 'Permanent Emergency,'" *Alternatives: Global, Local, Political* 31, no. 2 (2006): 191–213.

41 Barry Glassner, *The Culture of Fear* (New York: Basic Books, 1999).

42 Giorgio Agamben, *State of Exception*, trans. Kevin Attell (Chicago: University of Chicago Press, 2005), 22 (emphasis added).

43 The panel "Is It Time to Call It Fascism?" debated this question at the 2006 American Political Science Association conference in Washington, D.C. Participants unanimously agreed, with certain reservations regarding historical analogy, that it was time to call the contemporary political scene in the United States fascism. However, that is not the subject of this chapter. Instead, by the enormous risks associated with the state of exception, it becomes possible to treat the state of emergency with the attention it deserves.

44 See Carl Schmitt, *The Concept of the Political* (Chicago: University of Chicago Press, 1996), 26.

45 For more on this critical line of analysis, see Ashley, "Living on the Borderlines," 259–321.

95

46 Michel Foucault, *History of Sexuality, Volume 1* (New York: Vintage Books, 1978), 136.

47 Nikolas Rose, *The Politics of Life Itself: Biomedicine, Power and Subjectivity in the Twenty-first Century* (Princeton, N.J.: Princeton University Press, 2007), 64.

48 Schmitt states, "Sovereign is he who decides on the exception." Carl Schmitt, *Political Theology* (Cambridge, Mass.: MIT Press, 1985), 5.

49 Foucault, *History of Sexuality*, 137.

50 See Paul Rabinow, "Midst Anthropology's Problems," in *Global Assemblages: Technology, Politics and Ethics as Anthropological Problems*, ed. Aihwa Ong and Stephen J. Collier (London: Blackwell, 2005), 40–53.

51 Michel Foucault, *The Order of Things* (London: Routledge, 1989).

52 See Schmitt, *Concept of the Political*, 26.

53 Anne Caldwell, "Bio-sovereignty and the Emergence of Humanity," *Theory & Event* 7, no. 2 (2004): par. 2–3.

54 Ibid., par. 22.

55 Ibid., par. 6.

56 Amar Bhat, "Remarks by the APEC Health Task Force Chair," available at http://www.apec.org/apec/documents_reports/health_task_force/2005.html#AI.

57 Agamben, *State of Exception*, 29.

58 See for instance Ron Fouchier, "Global Task Force for Influenza," *Nature* 435 (May 26, 2005): 419–20.

59 Michael Osterholm, "Preparing for the Next Pandemic," *Foreign Affairs*, July–August 2005, 35.

60 To see how this materializes in Donald Rumsfeld's U.S. military, see Robert Kaplan, "Supremacy by Stealth," *Atlantic Monthly*, July–August 2003, 66–83.

61 See APEC, "Regional Health Threats," APEC, http://www.apec.org/apec/apec_groups/som-special_task_groups/health_task_force/apec_information_on.html.

62 Fouchier, "Global Task Force for Influenza," 419–20.

63 Laurie Garrett, "The Next Pandemic?" *Foreign Affairs*, July–August 2005.

64 Nelson Schwartz, "Rumsfeld's Growing Stake in Tamiflu," CNNMoney.com, October 31, 2005, http://money.cnn.com/2005/10/31/news/newsmakers/fortune_rumsfeld/.

65 Michael D. Christian, "Development of a Triage Protocol for Critical Care during an Influenza Pandemic," *Canadian Medical Association* 175 (2006), http://www.cmaj.ca/cgi/eletters/175/11/1377.

66 Christian, "Development of a Triage Protocol," 1378.

67 See Ong and Collier, *Global Assemblages*.

68 Nikolas Rose and Carlos Novas, "Biological Citizenship," in *Global Assem-*

blages: Technology, Politics and Ethics as Anthropological Problems, ed. Aihwa Ong and Stephen J. Collier (London: Blackwell, 2005), 445.

69   Ibid., 440.

70   See, in Ong and Collier, *Global Assemblages*, Gísli Pálsson and Paul Rabinow, "The Iceland Controversy: Reflections of the Transnational Market of Civic Virtue," 91–103; Sarah Franklin, "Stem Cells R Us: Emergent Life Forms and the Global Biological," 59–78; Vinh-Kim Nguyen, "Antiretroviral Globalism, Biopolitics, and Therapeutic Citizenship," 124–44; and Nancy Scheper-Hughes, "The Last Commodity: Post-human Ethics and the Global Traffic in 'Fresh' Organs," 145–67.

71   Eugene Thacker, *Biomedia* (Minneapolis: University of Minnesota Press, 2004), 5–6.

72   Ibid., 6, and see also 27–28.

73   Giorgio Agamben, *The Open: Man and Animal*, trans. Kevin Attell (Stanford, Calif.: Stanford University Press, 2002), 38.

74   Carl von Clausewitz, *On War* (Oxford: Oxford University Press, 2007).

75   Klaus Stöhr, quoted in Davis, *The Monster at Our Door*, 165.

76   Agamben, *State of Exception*, 86.

77   See Davis, *The Monster at Our Door*.

78   APEC, "Results From Survey—Pandemic Influenza and Preparedness: Situational Assessment for APEC and Western Pacific Economies Public Health Emergency," APEC, http://www.apec.org/apec/documents_reports/health_task_force/2005.html#AI.

79   *Fatal Contact: Bird Flu in America*, dir. Richard Pearce (Culver City, Calif.: Sony Pictures Home Entertainment, 2006), DVD. First broadcast in 2006 by ABC.

80   Donald G. McNeil, Jr., "In Daylong Drill, an Agency Tries to Prepare for a Real Outbreak of Avian Flu," *New York Times*, February 1, 2007, A14.

81   Paul Virilio, *Art and Fear* (London: Continuum, 2004), 75.

82   Quoted in ibid., 29. *Adbusters* magazine conducted a very interesting thought experiment in the summer of 2004 when it asked its readership to accept an end-of-the-world scenario and then report on life after the end. The hope was that, in those ruminations, people would begin to develop useful local strategies for the future. Note to the wise, although some reported that anarchy was fun, most lamented not having a garden.

83   Benjamin, "Thesis on the Philosophy of History," 257.

84   Ibid.

85   Agamben, *State of Exception*, 88.

86   Ibid.

87   Agamben, *The Open*, 92.

88   Agamben, *State of Exception*, 88.

89   Ibid., 87.

90   See Geoffrey Whitehall, "Viral Politics: Avian Flu, Difference and Con-
      tagion," paper presented at the 48th Annual Convention of the Inter-
      national Studies Association, Chicago, 2007; or Geoffrey Whitehall,
      "Infected Life and Viral Politics: Agamben and the Avian Flu," paper pre-
      sented at Canada Research Chair in Sustainability and Culture Confer-
      ence, Toronto, 2007.

91   For instance, see Cary Wolfe, ed., *Zoontologies: The Question of the Animal*
      (Minneapolis: University of Minnesota Press, 2003); and Cary Wolfe, *Ani-
      mal Rites* (Chicago: Chicago University Press, 2003).

92   Massumi, "Fear (the Spectrum Said)," 35.

93   Ibid., 36, 40.

94   See Keith Bradsher, "Global Effort Attracts $1.9 Billion in Pledges to Bat-
      tle Bird Flu," *New York Times*, January 19, 2006, A9.

95   Figures from Osterholm, "Preparing for the Next Pandemic," 25–26.

96   Bradsher, "Global Effort Attracts $1.9 Billion," A9.

97   For an equally if not more compelling tale of preemptive need, see Ste-
      ven Lewis, *The Race against Time* (Concord, Ont.: House of Anansi Press,
      2006).

98   Laurie Garrett, "The Next Pandemic?" 21.

99   Debora Mackenzie, "Bird Flu Outbreak Started a Year Ago," *New Scientist*,
      January 28, 2004, quoted in Davis, *The Monster at Our Door*, 102.

100   Davis, *The Monster at Our Door*, 102.

101   Ibid., 8.

102   Joint Chiefs of Staff, *Joint Vision 2020: America's Military; Preparing for Tomor-
      row* (Washington, D.C.: Government Printing Office, 2000). http://www.
      dtic.mil/doctrine/jel/jfq_pubs/1225.pdf.

103   Inspired by Chris Connery's comment that "resistance writes its own geog-
      raphy," quoted in Rob Wilson and Arlif Dirlik, *Asia/Pacific as Space of Cul-
      tural Production* (Durham, N.C.: Duke University Press, 1995), 6.

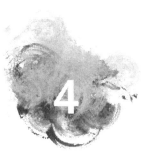

BIO TERROR

Hybridity in the Biohorror Narrative,
or What We Can Learn from Monsters

Priscilla Wald

Nothing has prepared the narrator protagonist of Jonathan Maberry's *Patient Zero* for the experience of killing people who seem to be the kind of people he would expect to encounter in a supermarket—"a middle-aged woman with lank blond hair and a stained housedress . . . a young boy of no more than ten . . . a pretty teenage girl in a short denim skirt . . . people in business suits and bathing suits"—but who have in fact become mindless monsters with voracious appetites for human flesh. Mistaking the smile of one of his attackers for a show of "relief that someone had come to rescue her," he is chagrined when "that smile stretched and stretched and stretched until it became a rapacious leer." The rushing mass is made up of victims of an engineered infectious agent that has turned them into mindless zombies, or, as Maberry's narrator says, "a predatory thing in human disguise."[1] The novel exemplifies a subgenre I call "epidemiological horror," or "biohorror," in which the conventions of horror meet the dangers of contagion, as a devastating communicable disease turns the infected into predatory monsters. In biohorror scenarios, the infected might seek to convert human beings or perhaps hunt them as a key food source, either compulsively and mindlessly, as in *Patient Zero*, or more systematically. The film *Daybreakers* (2009), directed by Michael and Peter Spierig, for example, features vampires who have ostensibly invited human beings to "assimilate" into the new vampire-run order, but it is difficult to accept the sincerity of the offer since the vampires require human blood to survive; their chief industry seems to be human harvesting.

100   Biohorror proliferated in the years following World War II, fueled by the increasing circulation and popularity of both epidemiological detective stories (often case studies from public health departments or the newly formed Epidemiological Investigation Service) and horror fiction and films. Toward the end of the twentieth century, a noticeable shift in biohorror stories marked a heightening attention to terrorism, especially in the United States: anxieties about bioterror in particular increasingly inflected the subgenre. The middle-aged woman, like the rest of the infected in *Patient Zero*, is, as the head of a counterterrorist organization explains to the protagonist, "the new face of global terrorism."[2] The marked proliferation of biohorror-bioterror narratives in such cultural forms as fiction, film, television, and video games over the past fifteen years (accelerating in the aftermath of the September 11 attacks) attests to the anxious intermingling of two contemporary preoccupations: contagion (specifically, outbreaks of devastating communicable disease) and terrorism.[3] The infectious agents are microorganisms, sometimes engineered, sometimes the result of military (biowarfare) or medical research gone awry, and sometimes the result of human encroachment on the microbe's natural environment. In all cases, however, the infected become agents of destruction, preying on human beings, that threaten to annihilate the species.

Popular cultural forms register the cultural anxieties and fascination that arise when scientific and technological innovations and geopolitical transformations introduce new ways of understanding the world. Fiction, film, television, video games, and other new media forms characteristically dramatize and, in the process, alter new theories as they appear in specialist publications and conferences and reach the general public through the mainstream media. New ideas circulate initially as a new vocabulary: images, words, phrases, and scenarios that quickly become conventional as they travel through the mainstream media. Popular cultural forms extend these scenarios by dramatizing them in the form of full-blown plots and interactive engagements. In the process, they act as magnifying lenses, amplifying the assumptions that inform the accounts offered in the specialist and mainstream media, thereby facilitating their inspection.

Monsters point to what a culture cannot (yet) classify and thereby embody the challenge to social categories that results from the circulation of new information and ideas about the world. The creatures that populate the proliferating biohorror-bioterror fiction and films have a story to tell about the particular challenges represented by catastrophic communicable disease outbreaks and terrorism, about why these perceived threats have become conjoined, and about the consequences of their conceptual entanglement.

From Microbes to Monsters

The monsters of biohorror narratives are in fact logical extensions of the microbe itself. For researchers, epidemiologists, and science writers whose work concerns devastating communicable diseases, the animation of the microbe seems almost irresistible. Microbes, for Richard Krause, "are not idle bystanders, waiting for new opportunities offered by human mobility, ignorance, or neglect. Microbes possess remarkable genetic versatility that enables them to develop new pathogenic vigor, to escape population immunity by acquiring new antigens, and to develop antibiotic resistance. [They are] more than simple opportunists. They have also been great innovators."[4] Madeline Drexler describes the canniness of their use of "a stealth tactic known as phase variation, hiding their immunity-provoking surface proteins and sugars to fool the body's defenses."[5] For Joshua Lederberg, that tactic "says they've got a memory. They're carrying about pieces of their evolutionary history in unexpressed forms, waiting to be expressed."[6] Laurie Garrett similarly marvels at their "ability to outwit or manipulate the one microbial sensing system *Homo sapiens* possess: our immune systems," and Richard Preston calls viruses "molecular sharks, a motive without a mind. . . . Compact, hard, logical, totally selfish, the virus is dedicated to making copies of itself—which it can do on occasion with radiant speed. The prime directive is to replicate."[7] These quotations are typical, and the tendency to animate the microbes in this fashion makes sense since the alternative is to accept the utter indifference of an entity that represents, according to Lederberg, "the single biggest threat to man's continued dominance on the planet" and whose "meat" is the human body.[8]

Lederberg remarks on the challenge of accepting "the reality that Nature is far from benign; at least it has no special sentiment for the welfare of the human versus other species . . . the survival of the human species is not a preordained evolutionary program."[9] The irrelevance of the human species is difficult to fathom; our stories put the species at the center of the universe (albeit differentially), the telos of evolutionary development, and the favorite child of Mother Nature. Human beings have developed the technology with which to annihilate ourselves, but no other species can pose such a threat to us—until we think microscopically. With all of our technology, we still know precious little about scores of devastating viruses and other microscopic entities, such as prions. The hosts and behaviors of microorganisms that cause Ebola and Marburg hemorrhagic fevers remain mysteries. As the language of researchers demonstrates, it seems easier to think of these entities as enemies and to imagine human beings at war with the microscopic world of the virus than to imagine the possibility of human extinction as the result of a chance event. In other words, it seems that human beings typically find it very difficult to imagine a scenario in which natural selection does not favor the species.[10]

Viruses in particular have captured the human imagination and account for many of the infections in the subgenre of biohorror. From the outset, scientists have been particularly intrigued by this entity that challenged conventional definitions of life. Viruses lie dormant until they encounter a host cell, at which point they harness its mechanisms in order to metabolize and reproduce. As new technologies in the mid-twentieth century enabled scientists to identify viral behavior, viruses generated wonder for the insights they offered into the nature of life itself. Awe bordering on mysticism characterized the earliest accounts of viruses, which appeared to inhabit a "twilight zone between the living and the nonliving."[11] In the most devastating of the emerging hemorrhagic viruses, the horrifically dramatic nature of the symptoms and the overwhelming infectivity seem to have increased the awe. As one renowned viral researcher notes, "Looking at Ebola under an electron microscope is like looking at a gorgeously wrought ice castle. The thing is so cold. So totally pure."[12] It is not unusual for researchers to resort to mythological language. Respect and even admiration overcome the fear of one scientist, who, staring at an unidentified entity with potentially species-threatening consequences, sees "white cobras tangled among themselves, like the hair of Medusa. They were the face of Nature herself, the obscene goddess revealed naked. This life form thing was breathtakingly beautiful. As he stared at it, he found himself being pulled out of the human world into a world where moral boundaries blur and finally dissolve completely. He was lost in wonder and admiration, even though he knew that he was the prey."[13]

The imputation of this mystical quality to viruses enhances their demonic nature, which is characteristically imparted to their carriers—or ostensible carriers. The ghouls of biohorror are the last stage in this process, which begins more subtly with an identification of communicable diseases not only with their actual carriers but also with those whose identity or behaviors make them suspected carriers. The identification of communicable diseases with immigrants, for example—typified in such characteristic formulations as science writer Barbara Culliton's depiction of "Seoul virus" as "another unwelcome immigrant . . . , a cousin of Asian Hantaan virus, which causes hemorrhagic fever"—fuels what Alan Kraut calls "medicalized nativism" and constitutes immigrants, strangers, or anyone identified as marginal or belonging to any kind of out-group as intrinsic carriers.[14] The anxiety invoked by carriers is amplified when an epidemic is associated with a particular population: gay men and Haitians during the early years of the HIV pandemic; Asians during the SARS outbreak; Mexicans and U.S. Americans (from the perspective of other countries) during the 2009 H1N1 pandemic. While there is a difference between being stigmatized and being demonized, the lines begin to blur, first with the rise of accusations of irresponsibility and subsequently when those accusations escalate into charges of deliberate infection.

The carrier has a long history of stigmatization and demonization in the United States, beginning with the first identified healthy carrier, the infamous Irish immigrant and domestic servant Mary Mallon, or "Typhoid Mary," as the media dubbed her. The theory that apparently healthy individuals could spread communicable diseases was still not widely accepted when the sanitary engineer George Soper first surmised that Mallon was the unwitting source of multiple typhoid outbreaks in families for whom she had worked as a cook. Her reluctance to believe Soper's hypotheses and submit to his tests and procedures earned his disapprobation and initiated his public depiction of her as "living culture tube and chronic typhoid germ producer."[15]

The identification of microbes as the source of communicable disease in the late nineteenth century and of healthy carriers in the beginning of the twentieth century fueled the public health movement and changed U.S. culture.[16] The ordinary social exchanges of everyday life became potential sources of danger. Objects such as library books, postage stamps, and especially money could carry disease, as could the stranger on the train sitting next to you or your most trusted friend or relative.

The carrier in particular presented a dilemma for the state, as early responses to Mallon demonstrate.[17] Because of her recalcitrance, she posed a public danger, according to public health officials, which warranted her incarceration in Riverside Hospital on North Brother Island, off Manhattan. But in the media discussions leading up to and surrounding her legal suit in 1909, the dilemma became clear; the state had an obligation to protect both the rights of the individual—which, many argued, Mallon's incarceration violated—and the health and welfare of the population, to which, argued others, Mallon posed a threat. The healthy carrier thus embodied a conflict between individuals conceived as legal persons (individuals endowed with rights) and as part of a population (bodies circulating through social space), which is also to say between competing forms of state power. The concept of the healthy carrier was therefore disturbing both because of the heretofore unrecognized health threat that such a figure represented and because healthy carriers dramatized the murkiness of the concept of human being and manifested its articulation as an expression of state power.

Mallon's construction as "Typhoid Mary"—her monstrosity—bore witness to this classificatory crisis. In her many roles, she lived the experience that Bruno Latour calls "hybridity," a term he uses to describe the effect of the artificial classifications that arise from rigid disciplinary distinctions. Hybridity results, he contends, from the "modern critical stance" that insists on perceiving the world according to the distinct perspectives of "epistemology, the social sciences [and] the sciences," which yield stark divisions between such categories as human and nonhuman, nature and culture. Those distinctions, which he calls "purification," obscure the networks and interactions that constitute experience. The many roles that objects perform as they circulate are fragmented by this perspective, making them appear to be hybrids. By contrast, Latour argues, these apparent "quasi-objects, quasi-subjects . . . trace networks. They are real, quite real, and we humans have not made them. But they are collective because they attach us to one another, because they circulate in our hands and define our social bond by their very circulation. They are discursive, however; they are narrated, historical, passionate, and peopled with actants of autonomous forms. They are unstable and hazardous, existential, and never forget Being."[18]

The newly discovered microbes of the late nineteenth century exemplify this circulation. In *The Pasteurization of France*, Latour observes that they were invented rather than discovered, which is to say that they filled a conceptual space that preceded their earliest identification. A communicable disease outbreak is both the consequence of the circulation of microbes and evidence of the social bonds and interactions that facilitate that circulation. And circulation is the carrier's sine qua non. When figures surface that call particular attention to that microbial hybridity, such as carriers, they embody the return of a cultural repressed (the artifice of classificatory "purification") and can therefore appear monstrous. For its role in elucidating the hybridity of human beings—their social and biological being—and in tracing the networks of relationality among human beings and between the human and the nonhuman, the human carrier is rewarded with monstrosity. That was true for Mary Mallon, the human "culture tube," in the early twentieth century and for Gaetan Dugas, "Patient Zero" or "avenging angel," during the HIV/AIDS epidemic, and it has continued in the depiction of alleged carriers—or superspreaders—in twenty-first-century outbreaks of diseases such as SARS and H_1N_1.[19] The appearance of monstrous carriers in the earliest examples of epidemiological horror in the 1950s and their subsequent proliferation from the mid-1990s to the present illuminates the classificatory challenges registered in microbial anxieties and their social and medical consequences.

In its earliest uses, the term "contagion" pertained as much to ideas as to disease and predated the identification of microbes by several centuries. Ideas and microbes often circulate along the same routes and by the same general means: social and economic contact. It is, then, not surprising that anxieties about contact and social or ideological contamination (the breakdown of classificatory systems) would find expression in fears about communicable disease. The identification of microbes enabled scientists to track the actual routes of infection, which materialized the analogy between the circulation of microbes and ideas (or ideologies). Better visual technologies offered deeper insight into microbial mechanisms and fine-tuned the analogy.

The rise of virology as a field in the 1950s, for example, coincided with an increase in the perceived threat of Communism, and an examination of the mainstream media and popular culture during the decade shows a metaphor exchange between the two. As scientists learned more about this strange, newly identified entity, they came to understand that viruses worked by taking over the mechanism of a cell and causing it to reproduce the virus. Viruses increasingly assumed the characteristics of Communists; they were devious and sinister, forming a kind of fifth column. Conversely, as anxieties about Communism came to focus on its propagation by internal agents, Communism increasingly became "viral."[20] In both cases, the agents of infection metamorphosed rapidly from viruses and ideas into human agents: carriers and spies.

The Cold War amplified both external and internal threats, reaching near hysteria in the United States with the well-documented fear of Communist infiltration. Popular magazines warned that anyone could be a Communist, and sensational events such as the much-publicized trial of Julius and Ethel Rosenberg and hearings of the House Un-American Activities Committee and the Senate's Permanent Subcommittee on Investigations dramatized the threat. Celebrities and neighbors alike could be Communist spies working to subvert democracy and the American way of life. Whittaker Chambers, Communist turned informant, regaled readers of the *Saturday Evening Post* with tales of "a 'sleeper apparatus'" that "waits for the future," warning that these "reserve unit[s] . . . will be brought into play only when those in control see fit—when events dictate."[21] Carriers who appeared "normal" could disseminate subversive ideas as easily as germs, and the two threats came together in anxieties about "bacteriological warfare."

While the nation assumed its role as a superpower and advertised its prosperity, the media constantly heralded profound dangers to its very existence that, as in contemporary threats of bioterror, seemed to lie at and even within its borders. The threat of bacteriological warfare intensified during the Korean War and was often paired in media analyses with the threat of atomic warfare. Both would result in effects that lingered long after an initial attack; in bacteriological warfare, those effects are the result of a unique and gruesome metamorphosis. Advances in medical technologies in the decades following World War II increased the possibility that engineered microbes could turn ordinary people into unwitting carriers—and therefore potential weapons of mass destruction—and quotidian social interactions into the means of delivery. The horror of bacteriological warfare lies in those perverse transformations, which have a double function in the stories. They manifest the porosity of borders and the regulatory failure of the state both to safeguard the rights of individuals and to protect the bodies circulating through space. At the same time, they display the *consequence* of regulatory failure and, therefore, the *need* for regulation.

From the vampires of Richard Matheson's *I Am Legend* (1954) to the undead of such recent works as Danny Boyle's *Twenty-eight Days Later* (2002) and its sequels, Maberry's *Patient Zero*, Scott Sigler's *Infected* and *Contagious* (both 2008), and Michael Spierig's *Daybreakers*, communicable monstrosity "purifies" microbial agency as it recasts it in more comprehensibly human terms. In Chuck Hogan's *The Blood Artists* (1998), for example, it is hard to distinguish between viral and human consciousness when a virus gradually assumes mental control of an infected environmentalist, who becomes a deliberate and vengeful agent of infection. The viral-human monster proceeds to seed epidemics of a virus of which he is the only survivor (if indeed he can be thought of as a survivor) throughout the United States with the idea of ultimately ridding the earth of its human infection. The researcher protagonists of the Centers for Disease Control and Prevention dub him Patient Zero—or just Zero—and remark on the danger of the transformation, "the character of a virus endowed with human traits? . . . We're talking about a being uninhibited by any obligations, social or moral. Combine the worst elements of a serial murderer, a rapist, an impulsive arsonist. Hyperaggressive, hypersexual, homicidal, egocentric, pathological. An unqualified sociopath. *The ultimate deviant terrorist mentality.* All Zero wants to do is infect, infect, infect."[22] Zero, if human, is a sociopath, but if Zero is a virus that has assumed control of a human body (an extension of what viruses do when they assume control of cellular mechanisms), then his actions do not make sense within human terms. He inhabits a "world where moral boundaries blur and finally dissolve completely."[23] Neither Hogan's protagonists nor the novel itself seems able to sustain that perspective. Zero is the "ultimate" in diabolical enemies: a terrorist who must be tracked and destroyed. *The Blood Artists* is typical of the vast majority of biohorror novels, which attribute malevolence to the infected even as they seek to depict the hosts as driven by impulse rather than rationality. The transformation draws out, as it literalizes, the subtle tendency to demonize the carrier—that is, to attribute the traits of the supernatural, animated, sinister microbe to its human host. Regardless of the source of their spread, microbes ultimately turn the infected into deliberate transmitters, enemies of humanity: bioterrorists.

Metaphor Exchange

The step from monstrous carrier to bioterrorist registers both a continuity with and a distinction between the early Cold War biohorror narratives and the more recent ones—between, that is, threats that resonate primarily with state and substate violence. In both cases, the monstrosity of the carrier is inevitable once the imputation of a microbial imperative to survive is recast as microbial warfare and the carrier's infection of a population escalates from callous indifference to outright malevolence, a result, as Lederberg's observations suggest, of the human intolerance of Nature's indifference. It is not surprising that a change in the political terrain will alter the metaphoric nature of a threat. "Microbes are a perfect metaphor for our fears" about terrorism, observe the authors of "The Infectious Disease Physician and Microbial Bioterrorism." The post-9/11 world, they note, "seemed *infected* with terrorists, unlimited in virulence, waiting to emerge from dormancy."[24] When, in a 2003 speech to the U.S. Congress, British prime minister Tony Blair remarked on the emergence of "a new and deadly virus . . . [t]he virus [of] terrorism," he summoned an image that has become, as Ronnie Lippens documents, familiar to the point of conventionality in political discourse.[25]

Conversely, for Madeline Drexler, "[i]nfectious agents need no visas. Secret agents shadow ecological change everywhere." Microbes are "nature's undercover operatives," capable of "hijacking the cell's metabolic machinery"; they even have their own mode of transmitting information: a "wireless communication system, called 'quorum sensing,' enables microbes to coordinate their activities."[26] Joshua Lederberg imagines the disease produced by our "ever-evolving adversary" to be "'Nature's revenge,' for our intrusion into forest, irrigation projects, and climate change."[27] *New Yorker* writer Michael Specter dubs avian flu "Nature's Bioterrorist," and flying geese visually metamorphose into missiles in the opening shots of *Fatal Contact: Bird Flu in America*, an ABC made-for-television movie that aired on May 9, 2006.[28] For Drexler, "the most menacing bioterrorist is Mother Nature herself."[29]

As these metaphors suggest, the terms of the comparison inhere in certain characteristics attributed to both communicable disease outbreaks and terrorist attacks, as it once lay in the analogy between viruses and Communists. As the authors of "The Infectious Disease Physician and Microbial Bioterrorism" observe, the near imperceptibility of the threat—the "dormancy" of microbes and terrorists (sleeper cells)—contributes to the similar anxiety they cause. Anyone can harbor dangerous microbes as anyone can be a terrorist, now or at some point in the future. Both make dangerous use of alternative communication systems and wreak havoc by corrupting information; viruses in particular work by harnessing and thereby corrupting the (nuclear) information that maintains healthy systemic functioning, while the vulnerability of communication systems remains a constant refrain in anxious discussions of terrorist threats. Communicable disease outbreaks and terrorist attacks threaten a similar structural, systemic disruption with the potential for social collapse as key personnel are unexpectedly put out of commission, consequently ending delivery of necessary services.

While such analogies are fluid, and therefore easily accommodated to a contemporary scenario, they also register the particularities of each term and modify it accordingly. The connection between anxieties generated by the prospect of outbreaks and terrorist attacks turns on the specific relationship of both to the state. The contemporary concept of "terror," although vaguely defined, is used primarily, as Susan Wright points out, for substate groups. As Wright documents, this contemporary concept of a terrorist threat emerged in tandem with the identification and naming of "emerging infections," such as Ebola and especially HIV in the 1980s, and both dangers found widespread expression in the mainstream media and popular culture in the 1990s.[30] Those depictions, which underscored the relationship of both terrorism and emerging infections to globalization and stressed the particular vulnerability of the state to its effects, increasingly came together, as she notes, in the threat of "bioterrorism."

Unlike concerns about nuclear war and espionage, communicable disease anxieties intensified following the end of the Cold War. Two factors in particular contributed to that amplification. The final decades of the twentieth century witnessed the escalation of warnings in the mainstream media about the exhaustion of natural resources and environmental devastation. The alarm had been sounded earlier, in the 1960s, in events such as the 1962 publication of Rachel Carson's *Silent Spring* and a 1969 report from the United Nations Economic and Social Council warning of "a crisis of world-wide proportions involving developed and developing countries alike,—the crisis of the human environment" that could endanger "the future of life on earth."[31] But such warnings found their main expression in the science fiction of the period, which often featured the image of the ravaged Earth's striking back ("Nature's revenge"). In the 1980s, the identification of virulent and mysterious new microbes—HIV in particular—exploded sanguine claims issued by the medical establishment about its imminent conquest of devastating communicable disease, which had served as evidence of U.S. cultural superiority. The threat of "emerging infections" brought the two factors (environmental exhaustion and the failed conquest of communicable disease marked by the HIV pandemic) together in an analysis that manifested the shift from a contest between world powers to dangers created by the very characteristics—such as economic growth and development—that attested to the prosperity and cultural superiority of the nation. The United States had grown so successfully that it had burst its borders: a global state that was ironically the ultimate victim of its own success. The shift prepared the way for the construction of the terrorist threat: the fear of violence associated with substate actors, often depicted in terms of a global network. The relationship between emerging infections as well as other catastrophic communicable diseases and substate violence lies partly in the state's implicit—and sometimes acknowledged—sense of responsibility for the conditions that have produced these threats, such as global poverty and careless development. That sense is manifested, directly or indirectly, in speculative analyses of both potential pandemics and worldwide terrorist attacks. It therefore makes sense to read the proliferation of biohorror-bioterror narratives—and their monsters—as registering the return of a cultural repressed associated with that often deflected sense of responsibility for the effects of inequities in the flow of global capital.

While Cold War biohorror narratives featured the corruption of channels for the dissemination of information, hence registering anxiety about an attack from within, concerns about the potential for that corruption have been even more pronounced since the 1990s, when alternative means of communication (notably the Internet) became more prevalent. The increasing role of bioterror in biohorror narratives has in particular amplified the horror associated with the perverse transformations of daily social interactions into the means of mass destruction, and the deliberate creation of *carriers* has supplemented the dispersion of microbes as a central feature of the articulated plot. There is a particular horror in the idea of infected individuals becoming literal agents of destruction in their families and communities. The scenario from Maberry's *Patient Zero* that begins this chapter emphasizes the ordinariness of the individuals who have been turned into mindless entities with insatiable appetites for human flesh and blood. The first team that is sent in to destroy them is slaughtered because these trained soldiers hesitate to shoot at the middle-aged women, businessmen, teenagers, and young children who are surging toward them.

The danger of that ordinariness is intensified when carriers are unaware of the status of their infection: people who do not know they are infected, such as the eponymous protagonist of Holden Scott's *The Carrier* (2000), have no reason to take precautions so as not to infect their loved ones. The initial lack of signs of infection maximizes their capacity to sow destruction wherever they travel, which the global ravages of HIV had made so devastatingly clear. Bioterror involving infectious agents, especially ones with incubation periods that last days, weeks, or even longer, capitalizes on the network effects, local and global, of communicable disease. It turns the networks of daily social interactions into augmented avenues of contagion; bioterror involving infectious agents, in other words, compounds terrorist disruption of state-regulated social structures by employing the very avenues of those structures in the service of (self-)destruction. That is the perversity of bioterror, but it also draws out a central feature of concern about the transformation of social networks into means of disseminating destructive information, microbial or political, on a global scale.

Microbial Transformation and Evolutionary Change

The nature of the threat of contagion lies in its mutual inflections of the biological and sociopolitical conceptions of collectives as well as of individuals. Microbes transform groups and individuals. Historians have demonstrated the role microbes have played in the outcome of wars, in facilitating conquest, in changing populations, and in shifting trade routes.[32] Given their transformative effects, it is not surprising that scientists have speculated about the role of microbes, especially viruses, in promoting human evolution. Science fiction and biohorror have variously dramatized that theme, depicting microbes as agents of profound leaps in evolution, as in Greg Bear's novel *Darwin's Radio* (1999) and its 2003 sequel, *Darwin's Children*, or Matheson's *I Am Legend*, in which the virus that produces vampirism infects the entire human species except for the protagonist, Richard Neville. Matheson's novella chronicles Neville's dawning realization that the vampires indeed represent the next stage of evolution for the species. Facing execution at the hands of his vampire captors, he realizes that he is "the abnormal one now. Normalcy was a majority concept, the standard of many and not the standard of just one man." Looking "out over the new people of the earth[, h]e knew he did not belong to them; he knew that, like the vampires, he was anathema and black terror to be destroyed."[33] This realization registers more than Neville's ability to see himself through the eyes of the vampires and consequent acknowledgment that he is an evolutionary anachronism. It also manifests his acceptance of the chance workings of natural selection—Nature's indifference to the survival of the human species.

I Am Legend offers insight into the nature of the anxiety surrounding catastrophic communicable disease, which entangles concerns about the social, economic, and political consequences of the disease with fears about biological consequences. It is well known that a major disease event can leave a biological impact on its survivors, as individuals and as a collective, not only in terms of a dramatic change in the population but also in the form of immunological and even genetic legacies. But the evolutionary theme of *I Am Legend* suggests a more radical biological metamorphosis. In his depiction of vampirism as a virus with evolutionary consequences, Matheson dramatizes the idea that communicable disease outbreaks are potentially "species-threatening" events.

As critics have noted, vampires and zombies, which account for the majority of contemporary monsters in biohorror narratives, represent different ways of depicting ontological anxieties. Marina Warner, notably, describes the undead phenomenon as stemming from the fear of the loss of the soul and notes the changing nature of that anxiety in evolving representations of the undead since the nineteenth century.[34] Biohorror-bioterror narratives show how the contagion anxieties that infuse terror discourse depict ontological anxieties on a larger scale. Harvard University's first professor of American literature once lamented that the influx of immigrants at the turn of the century threatened to "make the very name of us [Americans] mean something not ourselves."[35] Communists at one time provoked, and terrorists now inspire, analogous fears. Microbes, by contrast, have the capacity to effect such a change at the level of the species. If terrorists threaten to subvert an "American way of life," microbes turn the threat into a potentially evolutionary leap, which is, at least from the point of view of the metamorphosing species, tantamount to extinction. Lederberg repeatedly returns to the "Darwinian struggle" between human beings and our "ever-evolving adversaries."[36] Turning social transformation into a kind of extinction, the evolutionary inflection helps explain the often disproportionate sense of anxiety associated with outbreaks of communicable disease, whatever the source of the microbe.

That recasting also helps explain the monstrosity of the infected, who become the enemies of human beings in a Darwinian struggle that reaches absurd dimensions. Monstrosity, for Darwin, evinces mutation—a copying error that can be anything from a onetime mistake to the beginning of a new species. As Colin Milburn notes, it manifests taxonomic disruption and attests to the chance events that for Darwin mark change as the one constant of life; it demonstrates the fundamental instability of biological as well as social existence.[37] Milburn observes the centrality of monstrosity to Darwin's mythmaking: his story of human origins and collective identity that is at base an account of the intrinsic absence of origins and of species as an endless process of becoming, materially and definitionally. Microbial monsters in all of their incarnations dramatize how catastrophic communicable disease manifests multiple human vulnerabilities, from an individual's susceptibility to disease to the species' susceptibility to change, geopolitical as well as biological.

The evolutionary inflection of the monstrous microbes turns them into more than a threat to people. They also challenge, as they expose, the mechanisms by which a political entity is naturalized through its population. Michel Foucault coined the terms "biopolitics" and "biopower" to name the mechanisms by which the emerging liberal state of the eighteenth century justified its existence and exercised its power through the production of a population for whose welfare it was responsible. The state and the population are therefore mutually constituted with the existence of each contingent on the other.[38] When the biohorror scenario is the result of bioterror, the nation-state is typically the target, and it suffers a triple attack. The intended targets are the people (or some subset of them) and the political structure, but the evolutionary inflection means that the state and the population are also definitionally destabilized, with the consequent exposure of their circulation as "quasi-objects, quasi-subjects."

The evolutionary underpinning of biohorror and bioterror ontologically inflects the geopolitical and medical threats variously represented by terrorists and microbes. Certainly, that inflection helps explain the depth of anxiety, often bordering on hysteria, associated with these threats in the mainstream media and popular culture. The metamorphosis of microbes into bioterrorists turns microbes into deliberate, vengeful, substate actors and, conversely, casts terrorists as infectious, environmentally produced threats to species-being. Both pose threats that are at once material and discursive, and their monstrous hybridity contributes to the ontological challenge they present. They demonstrate, as they embody, the unstable definition of such terms as "human being" and "humanity," and insofar as that instability evokes evolutionary anxieties, it suffuses perceived threats to the state with the urgency of apocalyptic threats to the species.

Human Persistence

Biohorror-bioterror narratives characteristically affirm an intangible humanity that prevails despite geopolitical and biological threats. While appearing universal, the expressions and experience of that humanity are safeguarded by and identified with the state. As the advances of bio-technology proliferate, moreover, viral vampires and zombies increasingly share the genre with their engineered cousins: clones, chimeras, and other creatures of the biotechnological revolution. Featuring a clone rather than a disease carrier and a bioweapon that is a fictional dangerous form of radiation (thalaron) rather than a microbe, for example, Stuart Baird's film *Star Trek: Nemesis* (2002) offers an especially clear articulation of the state-species entanglements. The monstrous protagonist Shinzon was engineered to be a weapon of terror in intergalactic war; he was cloned by the bellicose Romulans from the Federation's Captain Jean-Luc Picard and designed to age rapidly with the intention of replacing Picard and fomenting revolution from within. A regime change on Romulus resulted in the abandonment of the plot and Shinzon's subsequent banishment to the dilithium mines of the Romulans' colonized planet, Remus. Taken in by the Remans, he survives and grows to lead a Reman revolution against the Romulans. The film opens with his successful conquest of Romulus and subsequent summoning of the starship USS *Enterprise,* which is under Picard's command.

Shinzon's motives are confused, as befits a monstrous hybrid; the entanglements that define him surface in a key scene between him and Picard, whom he is holding captive as he prepares to transfuse Picard's blood into himself in order to halt the accelerated aging process (and, incidentally, destroy his "original"). In response to Picard's query about why he is planning to destroy the Earth and the Federation in his quest for galactic domination, Shinzon explains, "It's about destiny, Picard. It's about a Reman outcome."[39] Significantly, it is Picard, in his response to this explanation—"You're not Reman"—who first manifests confusion about Shinzon's hybridity. Picard, in other words, cannot see Shinzon as having simultaneously biological and political affiliations. Although Shinzon has been raised among the Remans and clearly identifies as Reman, and although he is rendered monstrous in both of his identifications—as stateless terrorist (Reman) and clone—Picard insists only on his genetic (human) identity. The scene is informative for the slippage between these terms, as Shinzon oscillates between his political and biological identifications. He both explains (sincerely) to Picard that the liberation of the Reman people "is the single thought behind everything" he has done and angrily responds to Picard's dismay that he identifies as Reman with the assertion, "And I'm not quite human," followed by the anguished query," So what am I? My life is meaningless as long as you're still alive. What am I while you exist? A shadow? An echo?" While Shinzon verges on recognizing his hybridity, he nonetheless experiences himself as bordering on nonexistence. Shinzon, whose attire links him to his physically alien—monstrous—compatriots, is rendered increasingly grotesque as purple veins signal his accelerating disintegration and camera angles and lighting consign him to ever-deepening shadows. The furrows on Picard's brow show the consternation he experiences as he contemplates the implications of Shinzon's assertion: Picard can no more take credit for his nobility and heroism than Shinzon should be blamed for his appetite for vengeance. Since they are genetically identical, Shinzon explains, "you are me. The same noble Picard blood runs through my veins. Had you lived my life you'd be doing exactly as I am. So look in the mirror and see yourself."

The *Enterprise*'s android, Data, doubly rescues Picard, liberating him first from his literal shackles and then from the self-doubt and confusion inspired by his encounter with his clone. What distinguishes both of them—Picard from his clone and Data from his unremarkable prototype, aptly named B-4—is that they both "aspire to be better" than they are. With those words, the film refuses the definitional messiness of Shinzon's monstrous hybridity and insists on a definition of humanity that rests in the intangible (character, soul, whatever is signified by the ability and desire to "aspire to be better"). Shinzon's espousal of genetic and environmental determinism compounds his monstrosity and further justifies his exclusion from Data's definition of humanity. Ironically, however, that very exclusion implicitly underscores the hybridity that Picard and Data—and the film—attempt to disown. Any definition of humanity that excludes Shinzon is necessarily artificial and incomplete.

In its effort to reclaim a "purified" definition of humanity and reaffirm its intangibility and singularity, *Star Trek: Nemesis* is a characteristic biohorror-bioterror narrative. While the evolutionary inflection of microbial transformation underscores the instability of the definition of human being embodied by the (monstrous hybrid) carrier, the evolutionary struggle in these works typically metamorphoses into a heroic and ultimately triumphant battle for the survival of the human species. These narratives characteristically affirm human superiority and tenacity. Despite their superior strength and, in many cases, their apparent immortality, vampires, zombies, and other monstrous protagonists appear to be unusually unstable life forms, which distinguishes them from the evolved human beings of science-fiction works that explore human evolution. Devolution seems to be an ever-present threat in biohorror narratives. Even in Matheson's novella, while the vampires who represent the new world order are distinct from those that are truly undead (hence, more like zombies) in that they have developed a partial cure, they nonetheless rely on the continual administering of that cure in order to avoid devolving into their mentally deficient counterparts. In *Daybreakers*, a worldwide shortage of human blood causes the vampires to metamorphose into impulsive, violent (literally, bloodthirsty), powerful, but grotesque winged creatures called Subsiders. The instability in both cases suggests that the vampires represent an insufficiently evolved life form and implies that contemporary human beings indeed represent an evolutionary telos: everything else is devolution.

In most cases, human beings prevail, but in Matheson's novella and its first film version, Ubaldo Ragon's *The Last Man on Earth* (1964), Neville develops a cure but never gets the chance to use it. In subsequent versions, however, there are survivors who are either uninfected or who have retained sufficient humanity that they can benefit from the cure, which promises the survival and likely triumph of the human—and still superior—species. Like most apocalyptic narratives, biohorror typically hints at, if not outright insists on, human persistence and affirms the characteristics that fundamentally define "human being" and "humanity" as intangible, transcending any biological, social, or cultural terms. Monstrous hybrids proliferate, as Latour demonstrates, in response to efforts to purify definitions. In these narratives, they mark the unresolved conflicts and the dangerous consequences of those efforts.

Outbreaks of devastating communicable disease and deliberately large-scale violence inevitably register structural problems and geopolitical inequities and affect populations disproportionately. But the nature of the threats and the underlying problems are obscured by the ways in which they are being formulated. The biohorror narratives discussed in this chapter offer insight into how the naming and conjoining of the multifactorial problems of communicable disease outbreaks and substate violence result in their hybridization as the threat of "bioterror." Ronnie Lippens points to the proliferating tendency to depict terrorism as a virus since the events of 9/11 as evidence of the increasing medicalization of international relations and of empire generally, which augments the urgency of these threats and mandates an "epidemiological response." But epidemiological problems, such as communicable disease outbreaks, are themselves medicalized in the process, and the urgency stems from the entanglement of threats to the species and to the state, which distorts the nature of the problem and, consequently, predetermines the solution. As they offer insight into the medicalizing of both threats, biohorror-bioterror narratives can help explain how that process has foreclosed debate about them and limited the means of addressing them effectively.

In her statement "Return to Alma-Ata," published in the *Lancet* in 2008, World Health Organization director-general Margaret Chan invoked the 1978 conference that culminated in a declaration signed by 134 nations.[40] The Declaration of Alma-Ata affirms that "health, which is a state of complete physical, mental, and social well-being, and not merely the absence of disease or infirmity, is a fundamental human right and that the attainment of the highest possible level of health is a most important world-wide social goal whose realization requires the action of many other social and economic sectors in addition to the health sector."[41] The problems of emerging and reemerging infections and devastating outbreaks of communicable disease generally must be conceived of and addressed in social, economic, political, scientific, and cultural as well as medical and epidemiological terms. Nothing, for example, is a more efficient vector than poverty for the escalation of an outbreak of a communicable disease. The "purification" of this problem in medical terms oversimplifies it and thereby prevents the most effective ways of addressing it.

Bioterrorism, like communicable disease, has been hybridized as it has been medicalized. Disagreement about the causes of the kind of worldwide substate violence that has emerged at the turn of the twenty-first century is evident in the very debates about the definition of the term "terrorism." It is certain only that the dramatic increase in both the incidents and the destructive magnitude of substate violence, like devastating communicable disease outbreaks, has numerous determinants. Yet, the medicalization evident in the biohorror-bioterror narratives examined in this chapter shows how the tendency to construct bioterror in terms of human survival deflects attention from questions about how human beings live in the world: the nature and causes of political conflicts, environmental devastation, and socioeconomic inequities and their relation to both disease outbreaks and escalating substate violence.

In "Epidemic Intelligence," chapter 2 in this volume, Andrew Lakoff shows how the dangers of emerging infections and terrorism were politically conjoined in the United States; this chapter has sought to show their conceptual conjunction and to demonstrate how the biohorror-bioterror narratives register underlying connections among the existence of the state, the survival of the species, and the preservation of the intangible notion of humanity. Those connections supply the logic of what Lakoff calls "global health security," the anticipation of catastrophe and the safeguarding of borders that apply, as he demonstrates, to terrorism as well as to devastating outbreaks of communicable disease. As Lakoff also shows, reliance on the compliance of nation-states undermines efforts, such as the Alma-Ata initiative, that seek more just and equitable solutions to distinctly global problems. Analysis of the monstrous hybrids of biohorror-bioterror narratives can thereby offer insight into the conceptual work that must accompany these crucial efforts.

NOTES

1   Jonathan Maberry, *Patient Zero* (New York: St. Martin's Press, 2009), 236–37.
2   Ibid., 21.
3   These accounts represent one variant of what I call the "outbreak narrative," which names the circulation—in specialist and general science publications, the mainstream media, and popular fiction and film—of language, images, and plotlines that become conventional in a paradigmatic narrative about outbreaks of emerging and reemerging infections. For a full discussion of the outbreak narrative, see Priscilla Wald, *Contagious: Cultures, Carriers, and the Outbreak Narrative* (Durham, N.C.: Duke University Press, 2008). I am building on that work in this chapter.

4   Richard M. Krause, "The Origin of Plagues: Old and New," *Science* 257 (August 21, 1992): 1073.

5   Madeline Drexler, *Secret Agents: The Menace of Emerging Infections* (New York: Penguin Books, 2002), 10–11.

6   Quoted in ibid., 11.

7   Laurie Garrett, *The Coming Plague: Newly Emerging Diseases in a World Out of Balance* (New York: Farrar, Straus and Giroux, 1994), 618; and Richard Preston, *The Hot Zone* (New York: Doubleday, 1994), 85.

8   Lederberg, epigraph for *Outbreak*, dir. Wolfgang Petersen (Burbank, Calif.: Warner Brothers, 1995), DVD.

9   Joshua Lederberg, "Viruses and Humankind: Intracellular Symbiosis and Evolutionary Competition," in *Emerging Viruses*, ed. Stephen S. Morse (New York: Oxford University Press, 1993), 8.

10   A notable exception to this omission is science fiction, in which human evolution experienced as extinction is a common theme.

11   The phrase was used frequently in stories about viruses in the mainstream media.

12   Karl Johnson, cited in Preston, *The Hot Zone*, 122.

13   Preston, *The Hot Zone*, 197.

14   Barbara Culliton, "Emerging Viruses, Emerging Threat," *Science* 247, no. 4940 (Jan. 19, 1990): 279. Alan Kraut coins the term "medicalized nativism" in Alan M. Kraut, *Silent/Travelers: Germs, Genes, and the "Immigrant Menace"* (Baltimore, Md.: Johns Hopkins University Press, 1994), 3.

15   George A. Soper, "The Curious Career of Typhoid Mary," *Bulletin of the New York Academy of Medicine* 15 (June 1939): 705.

16   For a full discussion of those changes, see especially Nancy Tomes, *The Gospel of Germs: Men, Women, and the Microbe in American Life* (Cambridge, Mass.: Harvard University Press, 1998).

17   For a more extended discussion of this dilemma, see Judith Leavitt, *Typhoid Mary: Captive to the Public's Health* (Boston: Beacon, 1996); Andrew Mendelsohn, "'Typhoid Mary' Strikes Again: The Social and the Scientific in the Making of Public Health," *Isis* 86, no. 2 (June 1995): 268–77; and Wald, *Contagious*, chapter 2.

18   Bruno Latour, *We Have Never Been Modern*, trans. Catherine Porter (Cambridge, Mass.: Harvard University Press, 1993), 5, 89.

19   "'Typhoid Mary' Has Reappeared," *New York Times*, April 4, 1915, sec. 5; and William Hines, "The AIDS Epidemic: A Report From the Front Lines," *Washington Post*, October 11, 1987, X 1.

20   For an extended discussion of this metaphor exchange, see Wald, *Contagious*, chapter 4.

21   Whittaker Chambers, "I Was the Witness," *Saturday Evening Post*, February 23, 1952, 55.

22 Chuck Hogan, *The Blood Artists* (New York: Avon Books, 1998), 249 (emphasis added).

23 Preston, *The Hot Zone*, 197.

24 Sandra G. Gompf et al., "The Infectious Disease Physician and Microbial Bioterrorism," in *Microorganisms and Bioterrorism*, ed. Burt Anderson, Herman Friedman, and Mauro Bendinelli (New York: Springer Science and Business Media, 2006), 31.

25 Tony Blair, "Speech to the U.S. Congress on 17 July," quoted in Ronnie Lippens, "Viral Contagion and Anti-terrorism: Notes on Medical Emergency, Legality and Diplomacy," *International Journal for the Semiotics of Law* 17, no. 2 (June 2004): 126.

26 Quoted in Drexler, *Secret Agents*, 3, 8, 9, 11.

27 Joshua Lederberg, "Infectious Disease—A Threat to Global Health and Security," *Journal of the American Medical Association* 276, no. 5 (August 7, 1996): 418, 417.

28 Michael Specter, "Nature's Bioterrorist: Is There Any Way to Prevent a Deadly Avian-Flu Pandemic?" *New Yorker*, February 28, 2005, 50–61; *Fatal Contact: Bird Flu in America*, dir. Richard Pearce (Culver City, Calif: Sony Pictures Home Entertainment, 2006), DVD.

29 Quoted in Lippens, "Viral Contagion and Anti-terrorism," 18.

30 See Susan Wright, "Terrorists and Biological Weapons," *Politics and the Life Sciences* 25, no. 1 (2006): 57–115.

31 United Nations Economic and Social Council, "Crisis of Human Environment," in *Report of the Secretary-General on Problems of the Human Environment*, 47th session, agenda item 10, May 26, 1969, 4–6.

32 See, for example, Hans Zinsser, *Rats, Lice and History* (Boston: Little, Brown and Co., 1935); William McNeill, *Plagues and Peoples* (Garden City, N.J.: Anchor Press, 1976); Christopher Wills, *Yellow Fever, Black Goddess: The Coevolution of People and Plagues* (Reading, Mass.: Addison-Wesley, 1996); Michael Oldstone, *Viruses, Plagues, and History* (New York: Oxford University Press, 1998); and Jared Diamond, *Guns, Germs, and Steel: The Fates of Human Societies* (New York: W. W. Norton, 1997).

33 Richard Matheson, *I Am Legend* (1954; New York: ORB, 1995), 169–70.

34 See Marina Warner, *Phantasmagoria: Spirit Visions, Metaphors, and Media into the Twenty-first Century* (Oxford: Oxford University Press, 2006).

35 Barrett Wendell, personal correspondence, quoted anonymously in Horace M. Kallen, "Democracy vs. the Melting-Pot," *Nation* 100 (February 18, 25, 1915), 219.

36 Lederberg, "Infectious Disease," 418.

37 See Colin Milburn, "Monsters in Eden: Darwin and Derrida," *Modern Language Notes* 118, no. 3 (April 2003): 603–21.

38 See especially the following works by Michel Foucault: "The Birth of

Biopolitics," *Ethics, Subjectivity and Truth*, trans. Robert Hurley et al., ed. Paul Rabinow, vol. 1 of *Essential Works of Foucault 1954–1984*, series ed. Paul Rabinow (New York: New Press, 2000), 134–56; "Governmentality," in *Power*, trans. Robert Hurley et al., ed. James D. Faubion, vol. 3 of *Essential Works of Foucault 1954–1984* (New York: New Press, 2000), 201–22; *History of Sexuality*, vol. 1, *Introduction*, trans. Robert Hurley (New York: Vintage Books, 1978); *"Society Must Be Defended": Lectures at the Collège de France, 1975–1976*, ed. Mauro Bertani and Alessandro Fontana, trans. David Macey (New York: Pantheon, 2003).

39   *Star Trek: Nemesis*, dir. Stuart Baird (Hollywood, Calif.: Paramount Home Entertainment, 2002), DVD.

40   Margaret Chan, "Return to Alma-Ata," *Lancet* 372, no. 9642 (September 13, 2008): 865–66. Chan penned the statement for an issue commemorating the thirtieth anniversary of the International Conference on Primary Health Care, held at Alma-Ata, USSR.

41   Declaration of Alma-Ata, http://www.who.int/hpr/NPH/docs/declaration _almaata.pdf.

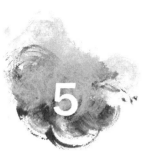

5

CONTAGION, CONTAMINATION, AND DON DELILLO'S POST–COLD WAR WORLD-SYSTEM

Steps toward a Haptical Theory of Culture

Christian Moraru

[R]*ather than morality or metaphysics, what we have today is an infection, a microbial epidemic, the corruption of a world whose predestined end is presumed to lie in good.*
— JEAN BAUDRILLARD, *THE INTELLIGENCE OF EVIL OR THE LUCIDITY PACT*

A civilization destroys another not because it is more "advanced" but because it has immunized itself against its own virus.
— DANIEL COHEN, *LA MONDIALISATION ET SES ENNEMIS*

We are embodied agents.
— CHARLES TAYLOR, *THE ETHICS OF AUTHENTICITY*

1

Anything but an aseptic proposition, culture originates and thrives in vivo. As we realize with unprecedented clarity today, "our" culture comes about heteronomously, alongside and across other bodies of culture. In all actuality, the problem of culture, no matter how immune to its outside a certain culture sees itself—no matter how strong its antibodies are or are thought to be—is the problem of the body in the sense that, always an incorporation, a corpus develops relationally, that is, in competition, conjunction, or, as the New Historicists would say, in friction with other corporeal agents. Culture does not become a touchy issue a posteriori, analytically, as subject to various (politicizing) interpretations, but is so from the get-go. Ontologically, culture is transmitted culture. It arises in transmission and remains transmissible. Hardly an intracultural phenomenon, it always obtains interculturally, by way of contacts, as it touches and is touched by other cultures, nearby or remote—as it touches on their themes, as it touches up their *Weltanschauungen*, and as its own motifs, fantasies, and conventions make an impact elsewhere. In brief, what touches off culture is touch itself. Touch is culture's *Urphänomenon*; these contacts and the ensuing influences do not occur between cultures already in place but constitute the very birthplace of cultural discourse, the premise of the most characteristic, culturally specific practices within presumably discrete bodies of culture. The Stoics were among the first to posit that while "to exist is to be a body," being a body does not mean simply being *in* a body, locked inside a carnal shell.[1] What puts us in "our" body by the same token places us in the wider world of bodies. Consequently, being in *a* body is being-with—being in the world, with others. As third-century b.c.e. philosopher Cleanthes argued, corporeality constitutes the keystone of universal interaction (*sympátheia*) both in individual bodies, where soul and flesh touch on each other by virtue of their shared materiality, and among separate somatic entities.[2]

Of course, "separate" may not be the best way to put it since the Stoic cosmos makes up a "sympathetic" ensemble held together by a "relation [of] mutual intermingling," and, again, bodies "intermingle" by virtue of their common physicality. Nor does this intermingling stop where political bodies traditionally do, at national borders, for instance. It is intrinsically transnational and transcultural, making us "all . . . members of one body."[3] Since, according to the Stoics, "one and the same nature has fashioned [us] all from the same elements for the same destiny,"[4] we all participate in the "*lógos* that draws everything together across time and space."[5] This holds true cosmically (we are one with the natural cosmos) as it does politically ("all men are brethren," proclaims Epictetus).[6] There is, accordingly, a cosmopolitanism of the mind, a philosophical project—rational, universalist; then, or perhaps in the first place, there is its flipside, the inherent cosmopolitanism of the body—material, contiguous—where immanence and transcendence collapse into each other.

Needless to say, Stoic universalism is not without its pitfalls. What I want to foreground for now in this *logos*, though, is not its universal rationality but an essentially incorporated rationality—"There is more reason in your body than in your best wisdom," Nietzsche intimates in *Thus Spoke Zarathustra*—more precisely, a bodily *relationality*, which, across and beyond Stoicism, underwrites, in particular, our dealings "in" culture and, in general, our dealings with one another.[7] Roughly speaking, we make and have contacts, keep in touch insofar as we are bodies. Conversely, our bodies supply us with encounter venues and communication tools. We have bodies, live, and develop our selves as long as we make contact and so live up to what the body structurally is. Thus, growth, successful physio-intellectual metabolism—the very narrative of individuation—boils down to an "infectious" narrative, to a relentless intake or incorporation of exchanges, negotiations, and relations, so much so that *our* bodies, which by force of habit we deem as fundamentally belonging to us and ending with us, representing and being us most intimately and exclusively, coalesce around and reference a neighboring heterogeneity: those "out there," not us. It is the feverish dialogue with these adjacent presences that our bodies body forth. The conversation would be unthinkable, and so would be thinking itself, if it were not for the "infectious" *páthos* of physical contact. As the Stoics assure us, there is no depth without surface, no principle without substance, no spirit without a body molding it, and hence no territory without limit and no access without its threshold and the trials of crossing. This is what Jacques Derrida stressed throughout his career and once more at its end in *On Touching—Jean-Luc Nancy*, in which truth, being, and selfhood are closely tied into the haptical (from the Greek *háptomai*, "to touch") and its themes: corporeality, finitude, liminality, and contact. It is in the ever-reenacted drama of contagion and exposure, in the contagious commerce with other bodies that we reach, he emphasizes, "a limit *at the limit*," that we go the limit and

125

thus, in extreme, geoculturally and epistemologically liminal situations, learn about the world and ourselves.[8] These bodies open windows into unexplored versions of the world and ultimately into the world itself as a whole, a *mundus* above and beyond whatever ties us down to our seemingly finite bodies, as Nancy says, or to the collective (ethnic, religious, etc.) bodies to which we are supposed to belong and limit ourselves.

"The greatest thinker about touching of all time," as Derrida calls him, Nancy builds originally, in *Corpus, The Sense of the World* and elsewhere, on the problems of corporeality and corporeal interchanges in Aristotle and Stoicism.[9] Noteworthy here is Nancy's case for thinking the complex, bio- and cultural-political thematics of the body over and against that into which the world's body, the *mundus*, threatens to turn as it is shrinking, that is, once it globalizes in the modern era of intensifying and multiplying worldwide contacts. For what Nancy rejects is globalization, not "mondialization." Published during perestroika, *The Inoperative Community* (1986) marks an earlier effort to envision a body politics for the aftermath of a Communist totalitarianism approached as ethnosomatic management—a set of policies, disciplinary representations, and practices regulating particular bodies and their mandatory, conspicuously limiting inscription into the nation's body. In effect, Nancy prefers "immanentism" over "totalitarianism," and this is more than terminological nitpicking. As he explains, in the ex–Eastern bloc countries, "private" bodies were pressured to "fus[e] into a *body* or under a *leader*" and thereby "expose [and] realize," "necessarily in themselves," the "essence" of humanness laid down by national ideology.[10] Posited as strict instantiations of the communal body, they were presumed to arise "immanently" instead of together with other finite beings, to appear rather than "co-appear" by rubbing up against other bodies in the world's shared space; they were not forming in relation—they were not relationalities—and for this reason they were not singularities either.[11]

The Berlin Wall's fall, Nancy points out, did not bring large-scale immanentist constructions of the body and body politics to an end, however. In fact, the stepped-up globalization of the past twenty years seems set on a "literalist" mise-en-scène of the Stoic "one body" as a oneness unmatched in world history. Not only is the world conglomerate of interlocking singularities, the world body as *bodies*, demonstrably more homogeneous today than before 1989 due to the growing range and force of leveling phenomena; it also appears to be on the brink of becoming a de-differentiated system, a "non-world." Bent on indistinctiveness, the world, Nancy alerts us,[12] is less and less of a world and more and more of an un-worlding world falling into "immundity" or abjection.[13] In his view, globalization has been parading before us since the end of the Cold War an indiscriminately self-centered totality in which touching equalizes those in touch and bodily configurations and their individualizing boundaries are disfigured, violently redrawn, or abolished.

2

Brushing aside the usual references to post-1989 economic progress and human rights in the former Soviet Union and its satellites, Jean Baudrillard contends, more alarmingly, that "the only thing" the Wall's "collapse released was the contagious germs of collapse,"[14] an assessment recently endorsed by Slavoj Žižek.[15] The last two decades, the French philosopher offers, have replaced Cold War divisiveness, isolation, and reciprocal quarantine of the previous alliances, influence zones, and of the people, goods, and ideologies therein with "the immense reciprocal contamination of the two worlds," which has in turn brought about "the automatic transcription of the world into the global."[16] In his assessment, the global "one body"—the world qua globe—comes into being through now generalized contagious contacts undergirded by *recursive* rationality. Inhering in a logic of contamination, this rationality, Baudrillard and others maintain, is a form of excessive or pathogenic haptics that results in cloning, metastasis, or, more often than not, viral outbreak. An epitome of the pathogenical, the viral is the haptical in its hypercontagious, repetitive form. Here, touching is no longer culturally productive. Instead, it contaminates by disabling cultural production on behalf of the reproduction of the same across the world's field of difference.

Thriving as it does at the expense of others, the virus is selfsameness par excellence and thus the quintessentially allergic body in the somatic imaginary of recent critical theory. For the virus cannot and will not bewith. It will only be: immanently and insatiably itself, ever the same. It will not change but morph in order to change others so as to replicate itself in their bodies, time and over again. Viral haptics is by and large one-directional. Ostensibly, viruses do seek out contacts; they do touch others and are con-tagious—"contagion," derived from the Latin *tangere*, "to touch," originally meant "contact"—but their touching is asymmetrical because little if anything touches them. They mutate strategically to sidestep real transformation. Reasserting each and every time the solipsist fiction of a body unto itself, absolute and absolutely self-begotten, their mutation is a repetitive ploy and thus, for thinkers like Baudrillard, a critical hyperbole that cuts to the quick of the networked society's cultural pathology.

Released one year after *The Inoperative Community*, the first volume of *Cool Memories* muses about global-age "viral revolution" apropos wire transfer, a banking method otherwise no longer revolutionary at the time.[17] Money remains, however, a typical instantiation of the overall de-objectualization and corresponding "viralization" of objects in modernity and of modernity itself. To move around the globe unhampered by locations and their borders—to go viral, hence global—money had to go through simulacral transformation and so became virtual. The simulacral, then, is the prehistory of the viral. Virtuality is the blueprint of virality. To spread virally, objects first de-objectify, lose their materiality and moorings in material contexts. As they do so, they turn into their own, self-displacing specter, the real's self-reflexively imaginal or hyperreal other. Hyperreality is the static infancy of virality, even though, via a reference to Paul Virilio's germane theories of worldly dematerialization and disappearance from *Pure War*, the initial installment of *Cool Memories* also remarks on the "virus of virtualization" and the "ecstasy of indifference" the world's simulacral becoming and virtualization bring on.[18] *Simulations* details this transformation's substages, but more relevant here is that, once completed, this involutionary process sets off pandemic multiplication. From object to its "deterritorialization" and de-objectifying representation; from there to the non-referential image, to the digital version that has little to do with the object;[19] and from the object's data-becoming, from its virtuality, to its virality, to its ever-speedier global distribution: arguably, this is a fair synopsis of Baudrillard's viral chronicles. I single out their last chapter because in it objects get "transparent," eventually "disappear" as objects, and then reappear, spectral, omnipresent and ominous, as pixels and computing code.

"Information virus" par excellence, the virus designates, as Baudrillard elaborates in the third volume of *Cool Memories*, "a communicable idea,

thought, ideology, image, notion or concept, that is created by someone, for no one in particular but everyone in general, which purpose
is to infect, seduce, subvert, and ultimately transmute the host society,
culture, metropolis centre, nation-state or any other system or cultural
circuitry, seemingly on a self-propelling redundancy overload that is
rushing toward its own collapse, destruction or annihilation, armageddon and/or demise."[20] That is to say, viruses communicate *themselves*, the
same information or, better still, the same *as* information. Vehicle of
sameness, they do not carry information proper. They are not reflective
of something or somebody else but self-reflective; they are redundant
and redundancy itself at work. The repetition they enact is senseless:
it will never make sense because it always makes, and thus has already
made, the same sense.[21] To Baudrillard, "objectual" modernity prized
originality and worshipped difference, the iconoclastic, the idiosyn-
cratic, and the idiomatic. Instead, viruses haul us headlong into a "radical
modernity" that, we read in *America*, "is founded on the absence of difference."[22] In the vortex of metastatic dedifferentiation, cultures bleed to
death—death as deculturation and indistinction. As with bodies, so with
cultures: "absolute death," the philosopher writes in *The Vital Illusion*, "is
not the end of the individual" but "a regression toward a state of minimal
differentiation among" entities, "a pure repetition of identical beings."[23]
"In evolutionary terms," he carries on, "the victory goes to beings that
are mortal and distinct from one another," yet "the reversion is always
possible." The relapse can occur in the "viral revolt of our cells," when
they "forge[t] *how* to die" and "g[o] on again and again, making thousands of identical copies of [themselves], thus forming a tumor." Or it
can happen in our "enterprise" of "reconstruct[ing] a homogenous and
uniformly consistent universe—an artificial continuum this time—that
unfolds within a technological and mechanical medium, extending over
our vast information network, where we are in the process of building
a perfect clone, an identical copy of our world, a virtual artifact that
opens up the prospect of endless reproduction." The "revenge taken on
mortal and sexed beings by immortal and undifferentiated life forms,"
from germs, viruses, and clones to Facebook avatars, this immortality is
pathological biologically, culturally, and otherwise, for it "actively work[s]
toward] the 'dis-information' of our species through the nullification
of differences." Equally viral on their micro- and macro-levels, genetic

cloning and globalization's cultural cloning "may well be," Baudrillard submits, a "deliberate project to put an end" to the "game of difference, to stop the divagations of the living," and ultimately to "eradicat[e] . . . the human" by setting up a techno-mediatic and mass educational system geared to making "singular beings" into "identical copies of one another."[24] Briefly, "we all have fallen victim to" a "virus destructive of otherness." A "site of the perfect crime against otherness," our "world [has been] given over entirely to the selfsame [*le Même*]." What with global culture restaging privileged bodies of culture, style, and theme, a wholesale "liquidation of the Other"[25] is under way, which endangers human togetherness in its relational essence by threatening to substitute "convirality" for "conviviality."[26]

3

Conviviality shapes life in late globalization more than ever before in world history, and it does so on a couple of intersecting levels beginning with existence itself at its most basic. To live and be "alive" (cf. the Latin *vivus*) is more and more to live-with (*con-vivere*). What I have said of culture surely applies to that which makes culture possible in the first place, namely, human life: to be alive has always been, but is increasingly today, to be with other living bodies, in vivo. Life too is inherently convivial. It posits the other as my sine qua non convive. I must be with him or her in order to be, for his or her presence affords worldly with-ness, a mundaneity structure on whose existence rests my own. This structure is, then, an existential-cultural form, an ethos, and an epistemological operator shaping everyday situations, artistic expression, morality, and intellectual-scholarly pursuits, respectively. It is, first, a form or material format of life insofar as it conveys how I am with an other in the late-global universe: I am in an unremittingly widening *geography of legibility*, in a world of challenges and problems whose solutions demand increased collaborative effort. Second, this structure is an ethos to the degree this reading-with, this joint venture in mundane legibility, calls on me to treat those I am and read with accordingly, as colleagues and peers. If the Cold War purported to break up the world into a mosaic of isolated bodies and buffer zones, today's world is one of adjoining and overlapping neighborhoods, an enhanced contiguity but also an ethical reminder that others have joined me in a partnership of equal footing, of fairness, empathy, and care. In a way, however, collegiality is a moral injunction already embedded in our collective venture in world legibility. After all, this is what "colleague" meant originally, the person I read with (see the Latin, *con-legere*). In today's highly proximal world, though, the colleague is more than an assistant or optional addition to what I already do or am. He or she makes my reading, my explorations, my discourse, and the identity coagulating in them possible. I read and am with so I can read, understand, and ultimately be, and because this kind of reading, understanding, and being is so vital to me, it behooves me to adopt legibility, the reading-with, not only as a form of life and culture but also as a responsibility. Stemming from co-reading-induced togetherness, collegiality presupposes a duty, lays down the with-ness law: *legere* refers to "reading" (*lectura*) as well as to "law" (*lex*). In a world become a world of vicinities, I "put together" my world picture and identity with an other, with my colleague, which brings me under the authority of collegiality as an ethical mode of being together, as law. This law "reads" ("legislates") that this self and other cannot go on reading—and, more basically, cannot go on—if, as they are and read with each other, face-to-face, they are not careful not to deface each other, not to disfigure each other's figures and meanings.

 A keystone of conviviality, the other's otherness is critical to the world and thus to our welfare. But, as Baudrillard warns, in the holocaust of virally displaced alterity, the world itself is receding, and with it the self's chance to come into its own. In Nancy's terms, the world's "ebbing" follows from the degrading of the *mundus* to globe on the heels of late globalization's cultural self-referentiality. This process, Don DeLillo too observes, is disproportionately self-indexing. "The world has become self-referring," he writes in the 1982 novel *The Names*,[27] and this is due to what might be determined as the "overhaptical," or the world's haptical overdrive; no more a world asunder, the planet has turned into a "near-circular system of rings intersecting across the globe," the writer told Anthony DeCurtis in 1990.[28] As DeLillo shows quite extensively in *Underworld* (1997), the two attributes are indeed intertwined. More to the point, self-referentiality or self-connectivity flows from *hyper*connectivity, which is an upshot of exacerbated, overly mimetic, and ultimately hegemonic contacts. A fallout of viral, "immoderate haptics," this repetitive excess is just that: too much, happening in less and less time, to the point that eventually nothing but the same things occur, or, better yet, recur, faster and faster. So what we are witnessing after 1989, Baudrillard and a whole army of critics do not tire of reminding us, is "the automatic transcription of th[is] world into the global,"[29] which is another way of saying that the language of contemporary globalization—the one language more and more people tend to learn and speak at the expense of the world's Babel of idioms, styles, customs, mores, codes, and so forth—is repetitive. Along these lines, the global—the world as globe rather than *mundus*—is construed as a cultural-linguistic pandemic, worldly expansion of a central logos or self-fulfilling prophecy articulating itself across and over other tongues and voices, making contacts with others but only to touch itself across their worldviews, vulgates, and habits.

This contaminating logos—surely not the Stoics'—may be intent on transcribing the world into global oneness. Language, however, does not merely repeat the already said; repetitive language—self-repetitive language, more exactly—is only one kind of language. Language, DeLillo insists, is also a "life-giving" force "shap[ing] the world" as it "break[s] the faith of conventional re-creation." In touching what it names, difference-grounded language ultimately creates—and thus creates its speakers too—*because* it opens up a time and space for others. This language, DeLillo avers, "lives in everything it touches and can be an agent of redemption, the thing that delivers us, paradoxically, from history's flat, tight and relentless designs, its arrangements of stark pages, and that allows us to find an unconstraining otherness, a free veer from time and place and fate."[30]

DeLillo's point on language and resistance to depersonalizing repetition brings to mind Walter Benjamin. "Even the most perfect reproduction of a work of art," Benjamin famously wrote, "is lacking in one element: its presence in time and space, its unique existence at the place where it happens to be."[31] However, "reproduction can bring out those aspects of the original" that we might otherwise miss or can "put the copy of the original into situations which would be out of reach for the original itself." For example, enlarged photos may show more, and more clearly, than their original; the camera lens may help us make out things the naked eye would not; and all pictures take us at least halfway to places where we may not be able to go.[32] Furthermore, the authority of the aesthetic object, its insertion into a specific "fabric of tradition," its inaccessibility, and its related "pure art" status and ritual-related "cult value" are all challenged, with positive outcomes, by modern reproduction mechanisms. Triggered by the latter, the depreciation of the actual artwork's presence is substantially offset by replication and distribution that bring the work before wider audiences. Mechanical reproduction has, then, an upside in Benjamin. Nor does it mean the same thing to the two authors. For the most part, "The Work of Art in the Age of Mechanical Reproduction" refers to the multiplication and circulation of a single art object; *Underworld* and, more broadly, DeLillo's fiction and postmodernism overall bear chiefly on the dissemination of a stylistic and cultural pattern, code, or form under the guise of "new" objects. The philosopher acknowledges the "auratic" dwindling of the original but considers it a reasonable tradeoff in a democracy of consumption. For the novelist, the main problem is no longer access but excess, not the public absence of originals but the overabundance of representations that, in setting forth the same things time and again, deploy a chronology of sameness where less repetitive formulas and designs are either brought into line or crowded out.

Hegemonic as this reproductive scenario may be, it is not airtight, which leaves room for alternate cultural haptics. The possibility does not lie outside the system of reproduction but is built into it, and *Underworld*'s network of potentially meaningful links allegorized by the world-system of waste at once conceals and divulges this alternative. If this system and generally the world are shaped overall by a reproductive logic whereby clichés and stereotypes recycle themselves endlessly, there is, or there can be imagined, according to DeLillo, a less totalistic, more creative system or counter-system of recycling. This works through and over what the "macrosystem" of production, reproduction, and consumption disposes of, and it also works counter to that system's material and political dispositions. This subsystem sets in motion a reproductive apparatus that scavenges with a difference, foraging through discards to recuperate lost meanings or lay out new ones. Where "epidemic" production is in actuality reproduction, this reproduction is productive, originating, as waste itself is or can be. This second-order production can manufacture its own aura: there is the authenticity of the original in the sense of Benjamin's modernist aesthetics, and then there is another one, according to which creation is not so much clean-slate invention as it is refurbishing, salvaging, working over, "painting over"—which is what Klara, one of *Underworld*'s artists, does—or "writing over," another name for DeLillo's own, consistently intertextual routine.

4

Redolent of the postmodern double bind that leaves artists no choice but to retouch the very stuff that touches their lives day in and day out, *Underworld* dramatizes the one-becoming of the post–Cold War world body at the same time that it disrupts this mimetic-repetitive process through aesthetic repetitions of a rather different kind. To be sure, *Underworld* enacts such repetitions as it reenacts post–World War II history. DeLillo zeroes in on both the macro-historical and the micro-historical, on the grand canvas of national and international events with McCarthyite witch hunts and J. Edgar Hoover's tantrums on one side and the minutiae of the everyday, the private, the neighborly, and the genial ethnic tableaux on the other, mining them all for embodiments of "unconstraining otherness." This is how inside the text's historical or, rather, counter-historical framework, plot-level counterhistories begin to unfurl, and so what DeLillo does with the novel as a whole artists like Klara perform in it. The novelist goes through the individual and global memories and memorabilia of the last fifty years to dig up specific yet unconsumed moments, and so does the character, in a saliently *mise-en-abyme* fashion. She recycles aesthetically—if quite literally—Cold War history by painting the B-52s decommissioned in the Arizona desert while "salvaging" (her own word) what was humanly unique, ethical about them: not the weapons but the life-loaded trivia such as the name of a woman drawn on a plane's nose.

Painting the painted plane: this is Klara's counter-painting of the historical canvas, much as *Underworld* paints its own, with Klara in it like in a campy *Las Meninas*. The planes, Klara tells Nick, were part of power arrangements that "held the world together" for decades.[33] Stretching across a "split" and the "curtain" marking it variously multiplied around the world, this togetherness was certainly spurious. A balance of sorts was maintained, though. A geo- and chrono-political standstill was achieved, with self and other clustered together around a semblance of difference but also around an array of effective distinctions enforced all over the world despite this admittedly oversimplifying polarization. Back in Hoover's day, the world was "held together," as it were, by division. The "connection between Us and Them," the FBI director felt, lay in the polarity itself.[34] Conjunction inhered in disjunction, actual or tactically played up like in *Unterwelt*, according to Klara, a "film about Us and Them" that staged the "contradictions of being, . . . the inner divisions of people and systems."[35] If Eisenstein "remade" Bruegel the Elder so as to put a human face on Cold War Manicheanism, Klara uses graffiti techniques on Cold War weaponry to "unrepeat" and thus "find an element of felt life."[36] The bombers and, she emphasizes, the "systems" the big planes came out of "repeated endlessly," standing as they did on a self-referential, apprehensive logic on either side of the divide, with "Us" and "Them" "spooked by [each other's] otherness."[37] The faceoff recycled into a panoply of ambiguously overlapping, private and public haptical "disorders," from Hoover's sanitary phobias of trash, grime, germs, infections, influenzas, and "outside" influences to policies of segregation, quarantine, containment, and deterrence.

After 1989, this *horror coniunctionis* of sorts flips over into its symmetrically excessive antinomy: the haptical frenzy encapsulated by the "fasten, fit closely, bind together" globalist mantra.[38] What Sister Edgar observes of the cyberworld holds truer and truer of the world as a whole: "[O]ut here, or in there, or wherever she is[,] [t]here are only connections. Everything is connected. All human knowledge gathered and linked, hyperlinked, this site leading to that, this fact referenced to that, a keystroke, a mouse-click, a password—world without word, amen." Logged in, DeLillo's heroine "feels the grip of the systems" of knowledge production and storage, the "paranoia of the web, the net," and the "perennial threat of virus" embedded in them as they lead her, one after another, to the H-bomb site. There, "she begins to understand. Everything in your computer, the plastic, the silicon and Mylar, every logical operation and processing function, the memory, the hardware, the software, the ones and zeroes, the triads inside the pixels that form the on-screen image—it all culminates here."[39] The bomb is an apotheosis of virality, but so are the bomb webpage and the entire World Wide Web. In them, rationality unveils its deep teleology or, Nancy would say, its "immanentism." Culmination—climactic contamination—survenes as self-fulfilling prophecy.

The apex is already in the first link and, before it and its html inscription, in the "primeval" digital input, in the initial "binary black-white yes-no zero-one hero-goat,"[40] which repeats itself ad infinitum like radiation and AIDS and repeats the world in its own self-repetition, writing the world's unconsumed moments, monuments, and sites into Baudrillardian "indifference" much like the thermonuclear tests blotted out "the foreignness, the otherness of remote populations implied in the place names, Mururoa, Kazakhstan, Siberia."[41] As readers of *The Names* and *Ratner's Star* will recall, this toponymy is a marker of the standalone and unrepeatable, of an otherness threatened by extinction decades ago and again today, when "intersecting systems" are "pull[ing] us apart" by "fusing us" with one another. So did the "atoms forcibly combined" in the 1950s warheads, and so do cyberspace links, for their coupling is nothing but "a way of seeing the other side and a settling of differences that have to do" with "difference itself, all argument, all conflict programmed out."[42]

A fully integrated and serialized system whose cut-to-size pieces spend their life cycles quoting one another, DeLillo's cyberspace is a post-differential, thoroughly contaminated world that paints a symmetrically totalistic picture of the late-global world. By contrast, Klara's project—and DeLillo's with it—is trans-repetitive. It recycles the humanness couched in the wrecks but employs the desert to block the recycling of the system in which the flying machines participated: "This is a landscape painting in which we use the landscape itself" as a "framing device" "unconducive . . . to industry[,] progress," and the other venues and narratives in which systems and networks of power perpetuate themselves.[43] The repainted planes may not be original in Benjamin's sense, yet they are no less auratic for that because, objets trouvés of sorts, they are not "readymade" but ready to use: they are "found" and then remade into something at odds with their initial meaning.

Underworld's "language therapy" is no less different. Under Jesuit supervision, Nick circles back to the underworld of "everyday things" to bring it out and thus build up the "fullness of [his own] identity."[44] This can be accomplished, Father Paulus tells him, through calisthenics that are no "mere repetition," through the "rote" that "helps build the man."[45] What the potentially artistic language of military discards is to Klara the "found language" of quotidian things and the commonplace is to Nick: a treasure chest of overlooked knowledge about others and himself and, more notably still, about others as guides to the fullness of the self. Tactfully Pauline, Father Paulus is quite adamant on the benefits of what he calls "the physics of language": to "produce serious men," one needs to develop inside them an *ethical space,* a "spacious quality" of body and mind that translates into "respect for other ways of thinking and believing."[46] According to DeLillo, this plenitude of being derives from a paradoxical heteronomy or studied incompleteness, which in turn results from an openness toward others, from the room we save "them" inside "us" so that *our* "ethical strength" can have a place to grow.[47] In the self moved solely by its own projections and appetites, this topology of otherness is under siege. Instead, DeLillo's narrative haptics both presupposes and boosts it through "de-ego[ing]" exercises that take us to the "spatial ethics" beneath the "spatial esthetics" of surfaces and its "autoworld of pain and loss."[48]

The exercises build moral stamina for they "repeat with a difference," reusing used-up language. "This is," Nick says, how you "escape the things that made you."[49] Klara, the "bag lady," poaches the thick-layered American and world waste systems to "unstratify the culture" and carve out an other to it; Nick raids language to make himself over and thus break out of the "hypnotic repetition" in play in copycat killings and copycat culture at large, in the "human presence"-free assembly line where his rental Lexus was put together, and in the "infinite regression" of the "endless fitted links" in the warheads' "alpha particles" awaiting mass-destructive self-replication underneath the equally repetitious "alfalfa fields."[50] He re-cites the already-said, calls it forth and out of the selfsame cycle of contamination. His drills help him veer from "the dumb sad sameness of the days" in which superficially distinct objects "collaps[e] in on themselves" to reinforce "the sameshit thing you'd said a thousand times before" under the pressure of "same[-]thing" entities such as "the state, the nation, the corporation, the power structure, the system, the establishment."[51] This pressure compresses time and space into "interval[s]" inside which things and people can be reproduced immediately—"serial murder," DeLillo points out, finds its ideal medium in instant "taping-and-playing."[52] This serialized reproduction is what *Underworld*'s artists fight, whether it is Eisenstein's "montage," the "scrounging" style of Simon Rodia's Watts Towers decorations, Lenny Bruce's stand-up, Ismael's "mural tagging," Wolfman's "bandit" broadcasts, or Klara's neocamp: they all stage repetitions that take exception to what they repeat.[53]

5

From Eisenstein's fictitious movie *Unterwelt* and its monstrous bodies tragically reembodied in the Kazakh victims of Soviet nuclear tests to the angelic holograms of New York freeway billboards to Klara's palimpsestic commemoration of "Long Tall Sally" on aircraft bodies to Rodia's acrobatics to Bruce's impersonations, and from the 1997 novel back and forth to the rock stars, movie directors, stuntmen, photographers, and writers of DeLillo's previous and later books, art involves, as often as not, incorporation or, better still, reincorporation. Regardless of medium, in DeLillo the artist is a body virtuoso and to make art is to metabolize: a body of work takes bodies at work but also bodies working on, with, or by other bodies, biological as much as cultural, which renders art making remaking and incorporation *re*incorporation—commemoration, intertextuality, recycling. This somatopoetics runs the full gamut, from Baudrillard's "senseless" repetition of cultural materials and the socioaesthetical contracts underlying them to repetition as production; from quantitative reproductions that rehearse the very "culture of reproduction of late capitalism" and in the process incorporate the artist himself or herself into the "sociosymbolic order" to qualitative reenactments that "avoid incorporation";[54] in short, from the iterative to the trans-iterative or transformative.

DeLillo's bodies and bodily practices illustrate these extremes and everything in between. In his oeuvre, some bodies respond to outside agents and more largely to the world of bodies superficially. Organically repetitive, they repeat themselves into indistinction and symbolic extinction. Bill Gray in *Mao II* (1991), Rey Robles in *The Body Artist* (2001), and Eric Packer in *Cosmopolis* (2003) are just three of DeLillo's characters who corroborate this repetitive model. Gray and Robles are artists who struggle to avoid repeating themselves into commodifying ("digestible") discourse, while Packer is a currency trader, hence arguably on the other side, and "part of the problem." They all end up, however, in the same place, the very place of absolute sameness—death—and their deaths are more or less suicides because their lives act out, with varying degrees of deliberateness, what earlier I determined as recursive rationality. This rationality is egotistic and, in that, assimilative; what recurs in its repeated self-reproductions is exponentially more of the same. Packer exemplifies this self-instantiation in mind and body alike. His digital models purport to predict digitality itself, repetitiveness—more specifically, repetitive phenomena in foreign markets—and he runs his body through the same routine day after day. He works out regularly, monitors his vital signs continuously, and is so obsessed with his prostate's slight asymmetry (an echo of Gladney's troubles in *White Noise*) that he has daily proctological examinations in his limo. But here, in the car on whose screens he follows the digital pulse of the yen and of his own heart, and, inside his extended automotive body, in his actual body, is where physicality reveals itself as the very rhetoric of consciousness, showing us, as an *Underworld* character explains, how the mind "looks," "what's happening" to it.[55] Accordingly, it is in the body that the logic of the selfsame jams, and this is exactly the point Packer's killer, Benno Levin, makes during their final chat: "The importance of the lopsided, the thing that's skewed a little. You were looking for balance, beautiful balance, equal parts, equal sides. . . . But you should have been tracking the yen and its tics and quirks. The little quirk, the misshape. . . . That's where the answer was, in your body, in your prostate."[56]

Levin is spot-on. The body has answers. As in *Cosmopolis*, it alerts us first to itself, but to itself as *l'Étranger*, as other: to the misshaped, lopsided, and twisted, to what does not confirm and conform, to the other-than-usual, and thus to the world's otherness, to that which makes the world tick.[57] "Suddenly it becomes possible," Paul Ricoeur wrote half a century ago, "that there are just *others*,"[58] and, still in Benno's words, our organs and limbs tell us, too, that "there is nothing in the world but other people,"[59] other fellow human beings and others generally: the bodyguard from the former Yugoslavia, the Romanian "pastry assassin," the Sikh cabbie, the little chapel Packer thought he could buy, the Siberian taiga's white tiger, the lonely shark in its tank, indeed, the world. *Others* are the world. And we must be with them—"an 'other' among others," Ricoeur also says in *Histoire et vérité*—so we can be.[60] Latter-day Stoics, DeLillo and other contemporary writers endorse this prescription by shifting emphasis away from the disjunctive and the confrontational, in which one body reproduces itself in, and thus suspends, an other, to the relational, where bodies morph into other bodies and thus gesture to overlaps, compatibilities, and affiliations that can be either reconstructed—they have always been there, are "organic"—or can be constructed for the first time. Either way, the body concept toward which artists like DeLillo work can turn into an other and thus latch onto otherness. For in DeLillo, the somatic matrix is intrinsically transcorporeal, a heterogeneous collage of body parts.

Lauren, the "body artist" of DeLillo's homonymous novel, is Klara's successor and, like her, "unrepeatingly" repetitive.[61] Earlier, I offered Spanish filmmaker Robles, Lauren's dead husband, as an example of containment of artistic discontent. Robles's first movies, reviewers claimed, paint "landscapes of estrangement" and other "alien places" where "characters are forced toward life-defining moments."[62] But since life in a mass-reproduction and mass-consumption society is substantially defined by a repetitive temporality at loggerheads with such non-serial instances, "his subsequent movies failed commercially and were largely dismissed by critics." "The answer to life" may be, as Robles declared, "the movies,"[63] but, one might be tempted to add, not *his* movies; it may supervene in a cinematic flash of "estrangement" and "alienation," but not if these terms mean what they do in modernism. If they do, and this appears to be the case here, the films drawing on these concepts are sooner or later isolated, commodified as oddities, metabolized commercially into socially palatable representations, used up by circulation, and finally discarded. Sanctioned by the death of the artist himself, the death-bound, public recycling of—"immunization" to—artistic insurgency is, *The Body Artist* hints, largely built into the avant-garde's "estranged" aesthetics. In it, estrangement and alienation boil down to unmitigated separation from those strangers with whom, authors like DeLillo think, the self must connect in order to make a difference politically, aesthetically, and otherwise.

Arguably, Robles's art is self-defeating. Not so Lauren's. Still a performance of estrangement, hers works, however, through and with strangers, through and with their bodies rather than apart from them. It is the stranger's body—Mr. Tuttle's—that plugs Lauren back into a world from which, after Robles's suicide, she stood disconnected, her body literally his body's "echo," "ruefully" retracing its downwardly spiraling trajectory.[64] Itself recursive despite its experimentalism, this course car-

CHRISTIAN MORARU

ried over into Lauren's own life and art as mechanical embodiment of the quotidian at its most repetitive and formulaic. "She tended lately," we learn, "to place herself, to insert herself into certain stories in the newspaper." "Daydream variation[s]" scarcely at variance with what they purported to be "version[s]" of, her imaginary conversations with these stories' characters or her desktop trips to the "dead-time" "[o]ther world" of the Finnish town of Kotka were forays into the ever-returning identical and thus into the atemporal:[65]

> You separate the Sunday sections and there are endless identical lines of print with people living somewhere in the words and the strange contained reality of paper and ink seeps through the house for a week and when you look at a page and distinguish one line from another it begins to gather you into it and there are people being tortured halfway around the world, who speak another language, and you have conversations with them more or less uncontrollably until you become aware you are doing it and when you stop, seeing whatever is in front of you at the time, like half a glass of juice in your husband's hand.[66]

Lauren inserted herself "between the lines" and into them, even "bec[a]me someone else, one of the people in the story,"[67] but, as with Robles and other DeLillo artists before him, this becoming and the conversations it enables were ultimately inconsequential. They failed to establish a relation—the strangers in the papers remained strangers—and for this reason, Lauren was assimilated into the media narrative, disappeared in her self-inscriptive performances instead of appearing in new, enabling postures.

Things change, however, courtesy of Mr. Tuttle, who shows up one day unexpectedly. More than any other character in DeLillo, he is sheer embodiment and by the same token strangeness itself. Possibly autistic, the boy seems minimally communicative, and his rudimentary intellectual behavior proves highly repetitive. Seemingly "just body," he is, however, an antithesis to Nancy's corporeal immanentism, for "he exists only in relation to other references."[68] He "is not himself" in the current, psycho-rationalist sense of the phrase, and as such he stands for an other to our notions of "normal," "functional," and "coherent" self. As a perpetual other to himself, he steadily backs away from whatever structure of selfhood is gelling inside him, so much so that his interiority exists only as a place where other selves make their appearance. He effaces himself so that they show their faces; he is solely in relation to them, his body a raucous "library" for words and voices not his but theirs,[69] not a link in a Lacanian chain of references but the very possibility of linking and referencing.[70] Purely relational, he does not engender discourse but mimics others' to the point that in and to him being is mimicry, repeating—not himself, despite what his name might connote, but others. To Lauren's consternation, he even mimics Robles's sentences and demeanor in an act of startlingly accurate if unwitting ventriloquism.

In the stranger's performance, Robles is at once himself and somebody else, but more important than the fidelity with which Mr. Tuttle "reappears" Robles is the lesson in somatic mimesis the boy teaches Lauren. This is a lesson in the humbleness of being as ethical "appearance" that does not do away with disappearance per se but, quite the contrary, is predicated on it. Disappearing does not signify melting away, though. It is a self-cleaning or self-erasure of sorts, which scours off the part of us that, in resembling too closely the images, stories, and conventions surrounding us, blocks out ethical contagion, namely, others' appearance on the stage of our self. Not only does this partial yet critical disembodiment clear the decks for Lauren's reembodiment performances; it is, in and of itself, serious body work: "This was her work, to disappear from all her former venues of aspect and bearing and to become a blankness, a body slate erased of every past resemblance." She cuts and bleaches her hair, exfoliates, applies rubs and fade creams to "depigment herself," uses astringents to remove all possible "residues," "dirt," and "impurities." More than "secretions" and "glandular events" of the "body cosmos," these are cultural footprints.[71] By taking in and embodying a wide spectrum of norms, expectations, and exigencies, Lauren's body has grown into a Foucauldian "microcosm of [her] culture."[72] If this growth has indeed stabilized and "rigidified" Lauren into lesser morphic ability by inscribing her body into the restrictedly performative symbolic order, what she attempts in emulating Mr. Tuttle is an artful regression past the symbolic and back into the semiotic and its unbridled performativity.[73] Cutting through the crust of cultural reflexes, Lauren steps beyond the body as cosmetic, superficial, and self-referring microcosm into the body as cosmos, the body as cosmic stage where others can appear. "Closing off" the repetitive order's "outlets to [her] self," the body artist retools her self into an outlet to other selves.[74]

Now, hers is "body art in extremis."[75] As Mariella, another character, comments on one of Lauren's performances, "Hartke is a body artist who tries to shake off the body—hers anyway. . . . Hartke's work is not self-strutting or self-lacerating. She is acting, always in the process of becoming another or exploring some root identity. . . . Hartke's piece begins" with a woman "gesturing in the stylized manner of Noh drama, and it ends seventy-five minutes later with a naked man, emaciated and aphasic, trying desperately to tell us something." "Alter[ing] her body and voice," Lauren makes her "body jum[p] into another level," the level or the world of alterity itself. "Stripped of recognizable language and culture," her body "flies" her various subjects "out of one reality into another" no less real, live rather than taped, across cultures and their boundaries of idiom, ethnos, and gender: a Japanese woman, adolescents, pentecostal preachers, "a one-hundred-and-twenty-year-old woman sustained by yoghurt," Mr. Tuttle himself and, in his voice, Robles's Spanish intonations and masculinity, which Lauren's body impersonates so well that Mariella "can almost believe [Lauren] is equipped with male genitalia . . . [o]r she has trained her upper body to deflate and her lower body to sprout."[76] The "agonic" theatricality of Lauren's female body works out connections with others—men, women, and a "number of nameless states" in between—who would otherwise remain alone and unseen, "in solitary otherness." The connections are not of the all-encompassing, impersonal, and impersonalizing kind, for their agony is "never the grand agony of stately images and sets" restaging themselves all over the world. Intimate and evocative, Lauren's "mysterious" body renders otherness "familiar and even personal" without serializing it, makes it less solitary by embodying it publicly, and at the same time shields its mystery.[77]

6

The mystery of the body and the mystery of culture: as suggested earlier, what we are dealing with is the same haptical mystery, the same issue of the body of and in culture, and vice versa, of cultural bodies qua somatic apparatuses. The distinction body-culture is, then, here as elsewhere, notoriously tenuous. Much like in the works of fiction writers and critics from Thomas Pynchon, John Updike, Joseph McElroy, Philip Roth, Kathy Acker, Karen Tei Yamashita, Leslie Marmon Silko, Mark Leyner, William Gibson, Bret Easton Ellis, Richard Powers, and William Vollmann to Lacan, Foucault (and Foucauldians like Judith Butler), Gilles Deleuze and Félix Guattari, Julia Kristeva (and nearly entire French feminism), N. Katherine Hayles, Donna Haraway, and Susan Bordo, in DeLillo, culture and the body are multiply and significantly isomorphic.

The somatic "images" how culture comes along, how it works and how it works on us, how it goes around, passes, and renews itself. Keen, in DeLillo's words, on the writer's market and on culture broadly as a "living organism" that "changes," "palpitates," "grows," "excretes," "sucks things," and "spews them up," this imaginary charts, in sum, cultural metabolism.[78] Given its bodily-biological implications, metabolism provides a fittingly dynamic allegory of cultural output, distribution, and exchanges. DeLillo and others like him picture culture as a complex, loosely systemic, and corporeal assemblage governed by ever-amplifying contacts and transformations and, conversely, identify bodies as symbolic sites of cultural action, re-action, and interaction less and less effectively served by modernity's pace and geo-intellectual maps. What these authors and thinkers canvass, then, is, on one side, the body of culture, culture as one body of texts, images, and sounds with their lives, deaths, and itineraries; on the other side, the culture of, in, and through bodies, the cultural-aesthetical constitution and cycles of human bodies. On the former, the culture into which bodies are born; on the latter, the culture a posteriori inscribed into them, made into, and remade, in and across them: the two sides are practically impossible to pry apart. Accordingly, turning to DeLillo as a case study in postmodern haptics, we have discovered that his viral narratives—stories of cultural making, remaking, and circulation, principally *Underworld*—document with rare acumen the workings of a first hyperhaptics, or "contamination," whereas the episodes of performative embodiment and bodily transactions in later DeLillo give center stage to a different paradigm.

Totalizing, self-repetitive, recycling the cultural-political codes and locations out of which it spins, the first paradigm speaks to the world as globe; the second, to the world as *mundus*. One is a symptom of globalization; the other, of mondialization. A mondializing world is still a world, more precisely, a *mundus*, because its haptic makeup—its self-touching, its overall connectivity—does not result in the kind of self-relation that bolsters only one self, thought, or worldview.[79] The *mundus*-like world is a non-totalistic *totum*, a whole where, while touching, mingling, and turning into one another, bodies nevertheless preserve their differential identities, as Nancy insists in *The Sense of the World*.[80] A plural, variegated *corpus*, *le monde* is a body-with; it is a body of, and as, difference. Within it, bodies converge, interact, intersect, and thus participate in the world's *totum*.

The globe's haptics is immanentist, metastatic—metastasis is "immanent," Baudrillard specifies—auto-referential, self-reproductive, and self-assuredly "rational." The haptic modality of the *mundus* is metamorphic, cross-referential and, in that, more "transcendental,"[81] humbly relational, and therefore productive—productive of knowledge, of new understandings. For the other's body is, as Barry Smart comments on the Levinasian "face-to-face," a face itself.[82] In turning to, and at times even into, others' bodies and corporeal structures, we face the face, the aspect of somebody or something of crucial import to who we are or aspire to be. This turning, or morphing, this *metabolé*, is symbolic. It is as much about physical and individual bodies as about cultural and political bodies, about national bodies and about the world's larger corpus. It latches onto biological bodies and their re-embodiments as metaphors of reaffiliations and transgressions that pull the "ekstatic" subject out of immanentist self-containment and into the broader world.[83] If indeed "the boundary of the self as well as the distinction between the internal and external is established through the ejection and transvaluation" of an "otherness"[84] originally constitutive of the self, much of the postmodern imaginary dwells so copiously on how bodies touch one another, on how they change into other bodies and swap shapes and meanings not just because corporeality is contingent, but also because it is profoundly contingent on otherness.

NOTES

1   A. A. Long and D. N. Sedley, *The Hellenistic Philosophers*, vol. 1, *Translations of the Principal Sources, with Philosophical Commentary* (Cambridge: Cambridge University Press, 1987), 7.

2   Cleanthes, quoted by Nemesius, in ibid., 272.

3   Eduard Zeller, *The Stoics, Epicureans, and Sceptics*, trans. Oswald J. Reichel, rev. ed. (New York: Russell & Russell, 1962), 136, 328.

4   Ibid., 328.

5   Michel Spanneut, *Permanence du stoïcisme: De Zénon à Malraux* (Gembloux, Belgium: Duculot, 1973), 14.

6   Zeller, *The Stoics, Epicureans, and Sceptics*, 328.

7   Friedrich Nietzsche, *Thus Spoke Zarathustra: A Book for Everyone and No One.* Translated and with an introduction by R. J. Hollingdale (New York: Penguin, 1969), 62.

8   Jacques Derrida, *On Touching—Jean-Luc Nancy*, trans. Christine Irizarry (Stanford, Calif.: Stanford University Press, 2005), 297.

9   Ibid., 4.

10 Jean-Luc Nancy, *The Inoperative Community*, ed. Peter Conor, trans. Peter Conor et al., foreword by Christopher Fynsk (Minneapolis: University of Minnesota Press, 1991), 3.

11 Ibid., 28. Also see Fred Dallmayr's commentary on this and related places in Nancy's work in "An 'Inoperative' Global Community? Reflections on Nancy," in *On Jean-Luc Nancy: The Sense of Philosophy*, ed. Darren Sheppard, Simon Sparks, and Colin Thomas (London: Routledge, 1997), 181.

12 Jean-Luc Nancy, *The Sense of the World*, trans. and with a foreword by Jeffrey S. Librett (Minneapolis: University of Minnesota Press, 1997), 9.

13 Derrida, *On Touching—Jean-Luc Nancy*, 54.

14 Jean Baudrillard, *Paroxysm: Interviews with Philippe Petit*, trans. Chris Turner (London: Verso, 1998), 9.

15 Slavoj Žižek, "20 Years of Collapse," *New York Times*, November 9, 2009, http://www.nytimes.com/2009/11/09/opinion/09zizek.html.

16 Baudrillard, *Paroxysm*, 10–11.

17 Jean Baudrillard, *Cool Memories*, trans. Chris Turner (London: Verso, 1990), 173.

18 Ibid., 30.

19 Ibid., 110.

20 Jean Baudrillard, *Fragments: Cool Memories III, 1991–1995*, trans. Emily Agar (London: Verso, 1997), 39.

21 Jean Baudrillard, *America*, trans. Chris Turner (Verso: London, 1996), 1.

22 Ibid., 97.

23 Jean Baudrillard, *The Vital Illusion*, ed. Julia Witwer (New York: Columbia University Press, 2000), 6.

24 Ibid., 5–16, 25–26.

25 Jean Baudrillard, *The Perfect Crime*, trans. Chris Turner (London: Verso, 1996), 107, 111–12, 115.

26 Jean Baudrillard, *Cool Memories II: 1987–1990*, trans. Chris Turner (Durham, N.C.: Duke University Press, 1996), 51.

27 Don DeLillo, *The Names* (New York: Random House, 1989), 51.

28 See Don DeLillo, "'An Outsider in This Society': Interview with Don

DeLillo," by Anthony DeCurtis, *South Atlantic Quarterly* 89, no. 2 (1990), 299.

29 Baudrillard, *Paroxysm*, 11.

30 Don DeLillo, "The Power of History," *New York Times Magazine*, September 7, 1997, http://www.nytimes.com/library/books/090797article3.html.

31 Walter Benjamin, "The Work of Art in the Age of Mechanical Reproduction," in *Illuminations: Essays and Reflections*, ed. and with an introduction by Hannah Arendt, trans. Harry Zohn (New York: Schocken Books, 1968), 220.

32 Ibid., 220.

33 Don DeLillo, *Underworld* (New York: Scribner, 1997), 76.

34 Ibid., 51.

35 Ibid., 444.

36 Ibid., 77.

37 Ibid., 77, 395.

38 Ibid., 827.

39 Ibid., 825.

40 Ibid., 465–66.

41 Ibid., 825.

42 Ibid., 826–27.

43 Ibid., 70, 71.

44 Ibid., 538.

45 Ibid., 539, 541.

46 Ibid., 542.

47 Ibid., 538.

48 Ibid., 457.

49 Ibid., 543.

50 Ibid., 571, 443, 63, 251, 458.

51 Ibid., 512, 711, 575.

52 Ibid., 159.

53 On "montage" and DeLillo's own style as both replication and critique of the "power structure it wants to oppose," see Philip Nel, *The Avant-Garde and American Postmodernity: Small Incisive Shots* (Jackson: University of Mississippi Press, 2002), esp. 97–107. Catherine Morley specifically addresses the influence of Eisensteinean montage on *Underworld* in "Don DeLillo's Transatlantic Dialogue with Sergei Eisenstein," *Journal of American Studies* 40, no. 1 (2006): 17–34. Despite the rather ill-informed treatment of Proletkult aesthetics and politics, Morley's account of the role played by Eisenstein's techniques in DeLillo's book is useful.

54 See Anne Longmuir's clarifying discussion of DeLillo's "two artistic paradigms" in "Performing the Body in Don DeLillo's *The Body Artist*," *Modern Fiction Studies* 53, no. 3 (Fall 2007), esp. 529–33.

55 DeLillo, *Underworld*, 511.

56 Don DeLillo, *Cosmopolis* (New York: Scribner, 2003), 200.

57 Jean-Luc Nancy, *Corpus* (Paris: Métailié, 2000), 11.

58 Anthony Giddens uses this Ricoeur fragment as an epigraph in *The Consequences of Modernity* (Stanford, Calif.: Stanford University Press, 1990).

59 DeLillo, *Cosmopolis*, 195.

60 See note 58.

61 On *Underworld*, *The Body Artist*, Klara Sax, and Lauren Hartke, see Longmuir, "Performing the Body," esp. 531.

62 Don DeLillo, *The Body Artist* (New York: Scribner, 2001), 29.

63 Ibid., 29, 28.

64 Ibid., 9.

65 Ibid., 14, 20, 23–24, 38.

66 Ibid., 19.

67 Ibid., 20.

68 Tim Adams, "The Library in the Body," http://www.guardian.co.uk/books/2001/feb/11/fiction.dondelillo.

69 DeLillo, *The Body Artist*, 86.

70 Adams, "The Library in the Body."

71 DeLillo, *The Body Artist*, 84.

72 Longmuir, "Performing the Body," 539–40.

73 Ibid., 541–42.

74 DeLillo, *The Body Artist*, 97.

75 Ibid., 103.

76 Ibid., 104–5.

77 Ibid., 110.

78 Don DeLillo, *Great Jones Street* (Boston: Houghton Mifflin, 1973), 27.

79 Derrida, *On Touching—Jean-Luc Nancy*, 53.

80 Nancy, *The Sense of the World*, 35, 62–63.

81 Jean Baudrillard, *L'autre par lui-même: Habilitation* (Paris: Galilée, 1987), 49.

82 Barry Smart, *Facing Modernity: Ambivalence, Reflexivity, and Modernity* (London: Sage, 1999), 124–30.

83 On Nancy's "'ekstatic' self-transgression," see Dallmayr, "An 'Inoperative' Global Community?" 178.

84 Judith Butler, *Gender Trouble: Feminism and the Subversion of Identity* (New York: Routledge, 1999), 170.

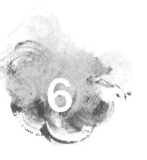

CONTAGION OF INTELLECTUAL TRADITIONS IN POST-9/11 NOVELS

Alberto S. Galindo

I want your ugly.
I want your disease.
I want your everything
As long as it's free.
— LADY GAGA

Judith Butler's 2004 essay collection *Precarious Life* opens with a clear and strong condemnation of post-9/11 censorship and anti-intellectualism.[1] In relation to Butler's suggestive hypotheses, this chapter explores the ways in which two post-9/11 fiction works in prose try to comment on, evade, or outwit governmental and imperial mechanisms of a discourse against an open and intellectual debate in a post-9/11 United States.

The chapter brings together an American writer's novel, Claire Messud's *The Emperor Children* (2006), and a novel by a British writer, Zoë Heller's *The Believers* (2009). Both novels are threaded by the socioeconomic privilege that their respective characters have and the luxury that such freedom affords them when dealing with, coping with, and surviving the events of September 11 and their aftermath. Most of the main characters in these two novels form their narratives from the class position that the character Rosa in *The Believers* calls "bourgeois liberalism."[2] It is this bourgeois liberalism that becomes one of the central ideologies in both novels and then spreads metaphorically throughout the texts, similar to the spread of Communism as a metaphor of contagion during the Cold War.[3] Thus, this chapter explores not the literal, bodily notion of contagion but rather the contagion of intellectual ideas, primarily the characters' constant implicit and explicit acceptance of a bourgeois notion of liberalism in the aftermath of 9/11.

The choice of two women writers and their nationalities is not serendipitous. It is, partly, a response to the observations made by scholars and critics such as Kristiaan Versluys, who writes: "It is also a matter of mere conjecture whether the new 9/11 fiction will remain the preserve of male white writers or whether it will be marked by more gender and ethnic diversity or acquire a more outspoken international dimension."[4]

Besides the common ground both writers share, the novels are both third-person narratives concerned with the bonds and ties of bourgeois liberal families who are affected by the events of 9/11, and this, in turn, generates a fictional dialogue between the politics of both texts.[5]

Emerging from a character's notion of bourgeois liberalism, this chapter also invokes the concept of ideology constructed in the novel through a digested version that several characters conceive based on some of Antonio Gramsci's writings. The ideological apparatus is derived from and referenced by, in the case of *The Believers*, a famous quote attributed to Gramsci that serves as the epigraph to Heller's novel: "The challenge of modernity is to live without illusions and without becoming disillusioned." The scope of a bourgeois liberalism and its hegemonic culture clearly expands through the texts in contrast or response to ideological premises that are feared and criticized by the characters in the present, such as Rosa's previous interest in communist socialism, but that may have marked their lives in the past, as in the case of the patriarch in *The Believers*, who claims that his epitaph will be by Gramsci as well: "a pessimist because of intelligence and an optimist by will."[6] The privilege of these characters in *The Believers*, who quote Gramsci at will,

creates an environment that allows for the construction of subtle metaphors of contagion, or social contagion as studied by sociologists.[7] It is
the epigraph's question of modernity and illusions that permeates the
characters in *The Believers*, but also in *The Emperor's Children*, especially if
seen through Gramsci's notion that ideology—the bourgeois liberalism
mentioned here as well as the culture indispensable to maintaining such
liberalism—does create these characters and provoke them to act. Such
political and intellectual action can be read in the novels particularly
because both texts push for public intellectuals or figures who try to take
charge of ideological practices and their respective intellectual debates.[8]

The characters in *The Emperor's Children* fear the anti-intellectualism
and censorship that Butler studies in *Precarious Life*, and in order to avoid
these, they want to spread intellectualism, in its privileged and bourgeois
version. The response to their concern with this metaphoric contagion is
to generate and speak from another form of contagion, but without perceiving it in such a way. In their attempts to counteract the expansion of
one form of contagious, neoliberal cultural stagnation, they participate
willingly in another iteration of metaphoric contagion, namely, a liberal
cultural revolution in this case. These characters, as well as most in *The
Believers*, desire and engage with a contagious bourgeois liberalism that
they hope will spread like contagious laughter. This chapter focuses on
the pacts these characters have made with their respective ideologies and
the ways in which such ideologies become metaphors of wishful contagion that spread throughout these fictions.

If, on the one hand, both novels can be tied to questions of ideology
through the use and reading of Gramsci in the text of *The Believers*, then,
on the other, the following epigraph in *The Emperor's Children* suggests
issues surrounding the use and construction of narratives: "The General, speaking one felt with authority, always insisted that, if you bring
off adequate preservation of your personal myth, nothing much else in
life matters. It is not what happens to people that is significant, but what
they think happens to them." The quote, from Anthony Powell's 1971
novel *Books Do Furnish a Room*, allows Messud to introduce the question
of narrative, especially in the form of myth, while simultaneously allud-
ing to Powell's interest in humor in literature, especially satire. These
two epigraphs, from Gramsci and Powell, guide the construction of both
novels as well as the reading proposed by this chapter: the turns in the

narrative form in relation to the ideology of a bourgeois liberalism that spreads through the novels in metaphoric ways.

These metaphors arise from two different post-9/11 moments, 2006 and 2009, in order to remind us that "our understanding of September 11 is incremental and can never hope to be intact and entire," as Martin Amis claims in his introductory note to his collection of stories and essays *The Second Plane*.[9] These post-9/11 moments are present both in fiction and in some literary criticism of post-9/11 novels that has been instrumental in questioning the narrative and thematic questions raised in these texts as well as in in generating its own critical discourse for the analysis of this literature. Richard Gray creates a brief yet substantial genealogy in his essay "American Prose Writing at a Time of Crisis," in which he explores some well-known post-9/11 novels. Gray makes three crucial points. First, he clearly states that the novels he is analyzing are marked by the narration and theoretical framework of trauma theory[10] and even claims such narratives fail at exploring any post-9/11 complexities because they are indeed focused on the trauma of a post-9/11 United States.[11] His second significant point is centered on the narrative form itself as he claims that these novels rely on a form that may not allow for any kind of insightful narration. Gray's final observation turns into a prescription for post-9/11 novelists, almost requiring that this literature should become *deterritorialized*—borrowing from Deleuze and Guattari—while focusing on immigrant narratives. For Gray, in other words, the questions that post-9/11 fiction must ask should arise from dislocating commonplace post-9/11 narrative voices (meaning mostly those of white, privileged characters) from their national territory (meaning mostly a white, privileged United States). The shortfall of his recommendation is clearly explored in Michael Rothberg's response to Gray in the same issue of *American Literary History*.[12] Rothberg states that the politics of a *deterritorialized*, immigrant literature can indeed constitute a sharp point of entry into 9/11 in the United States, but he also prescribes that post-9/11 fiction not only be about the United States; this fiction, according to Rothberg, should also be about the effects of the United States on other countries. If both prescriptions are joined together, it seems that Gray and Rothberg are asking for an American Franz Kafka, a writer who could produce texts of what Deleuze and Guattari term "minor literature": a political literature of collective value written in the language of the majority but from a marginal or marginalized position.[13] This kind of writer would exemplify the kind of narrative decentralization that Butler calls for in *Precarious Life*. It should be noted, however, that Rothberg's response uses an example of literature that is not American; he goes to *Netherland* (2008) by Joseph O'Neill, an Irishman raised in Holland, in order to establish a contrast with the American novels that Gray studies, including those by canonical writers such as Don DeLillo, Cormac McCarthy, and John Updike.

This chapter also seeks to dialogue with Gray's and Rothberg's recommendations for post-9/11 novels, not in order to explore the points that some of this literature fails to accomplish or address, but rather to address the issues that this literature seems to be putting forward.

The Emperor's Children and the Question of Timing

Claire Messud's novel *The Emperor's Children* spends most of its pages, its first forty-six short chapters, in a pre-9/11 world, slowly presenting its characters in March, May, and July of 2001 until their lives are marked by September 11 in chapter fifty-eight. The chapter "The Morning After" presents Murray Thwaite, a public intellectual and journalist, stuck in a Lower Manhattan apartment with his mistress, Danielle, while his wife thinks he is in Chicago. On this morning of crisis, he decides to walk uptown to his wife and apartment while leaving his mistress behind. Danielle experiences the chaos of the day only in a personal way, from the perspective of the jilted lover. Her concerns center on her own situation; it is not about collective injury or collective trauma but rather the surprise, the shock of a relationship that has ended because of 9/11.[14] This day does change everything for Danielle, for she understands that Murray will be shaken and will reconcile with his wife. Danielle is the first character in Messud's novel to experience the morning of September 11. She is aware that perhaps she should step away from the private sphere and enter the realm of the public "because in the light of these things she did not matter,"[15] but for her, 9/11 is the end of her future with Murray. And 9/11 will continue to represent that end for her throughout the rest of the novel.

The next chapter presents the opposite of Danielle's notion of 9/11 as a situation in the private sphere by focusing on the reaction of her lover's daughter, Marina Thwaite, and Marina's husband, Ludovic. Ludovic suggests that he and Marina should immediately leave the offices of the magazine they are about to launch, and Marina responds by asking if they should walk on the streets because they have a responsibility as journalists. He replies that they should be outside because history is unfolding and they cannot pretend otherwise. Outside the office, criticism of the immediate response to 9/11 comes via Ludovic, the foreigner who came to the United States to found and edit *The Monitor*, a political magazine. They walk around Union Square for a while, and he reacts to posters of people who are missing after the Twin Towers' collapse by hyperbolically calling such posters "necrophiliac pornography."[16] Ludovic is the one character afforded the opportunity to express a critical perspective on 9/11 solidarity, concern, or grief, mostly because he will never risk being called un-American or unpatriotic because he is foreign. The anti-intellectualism Marina and Ludovic fear, that is, the background premise for *The Monitor*'s launch, instantly gains even more force on September 11. Hoping to offset the metaphoric contagion of pre- and post-9/11 anti-intellectualism, they want to disseminate a contagious, leftist, bourgeois liberalism through the costly publication of a political magazine.

The question of being American or un-American is phrased more directly after the members of the Thwaite family find themselves in an uncertain situation when they discover that Frederick "Bootie" Tubb, Murray's nephew and Judy Thwaite's son, has gone missing. Marina and her friend, Julius, go to Fort Greene, Brooklyn, to search for Bootie at his place since his mother lives upstate. Once they arrive, Julius focuses on the value of real estate in the area: "If I had a million, I'd buy this dump and do it up. Sooner or later, it's going to be worth a lot."[17] Marina not only agrees with this observation but also confesses to having noticed the same in the block they have just passed. Marina had reacted negatively to Ludovic's description of post-9/11 New York as "necrophiliac pornography" but finds herself in a position to comment on real estate potential just a couple of days after the events, again reenacting their world of socioeconomic privilege or "First World complacency," to borrow again from Butler's text.[18] They may not have the actual money to "buy this dump and do it up," but they clearly speak from that position, which brings to mind the speech President George W. Bush made on September 20, 2001: "I ask your continued participation and confidence in the American economy. Terrorists attacked a symbol of American prosperity; they did not touch its source."[19] Marina and Julius, in this minor exchange, clearly exemplify the acts that the president would soon advocate. *The Emperor's Children* then uses Bootie's disappearance as a mechanism for reflecting on American prosperity, as suggested by the fictional characters as well as the historical president.

With 9/11 comes the end of *The Monitor*. The head financier behind *The Monitor* explains that "nobody wanted such a thing in this new world, a frivolous, satirical thing." These characters in New York, in the immediacy of 9/11, are aware of the heavy seriousness of these events and the reduced role, if any, of any sort of humor in commenting instantly on 9/11. The novel seems to enter into dialogue with the unhesitant declaration of the end of irony made immediately after 9/11 by many public figures such as Graydon Carter of *Vanity Fair* and Roger Rosenblatt of *Time* magazine.[20] The description of *The Monitor* as a work of satire seems crucial here, especially in the context of post-9/11 debates on the uses and abuses of humor. Parts of this debate have been summed up by Amis, for example, as follows: "Islam, as I said, is a total system, and like such systems it is eerily amenable to satire. But with Islamism, with total malignancy, with total terror and total boredom, irony, even militant irony (which is what satire is), merely shrivels and dies"[21]

Within the novel, there are two crucial moments of irony that perhaps allow for some intellectual distance from 9/11. The turn of the screw in *The Emperor's Children* is the way in which Bootie uses the day advantageously. Every member of the Thwaite family, including his mother, uncle, and cousin, have been looking incessantly for news about him, but, as it turns out, he has taken a bus down to Florida.[22] Bootie consciously does the almost unspeakable: he wants to disappear by allowing everyone else to think he has died; he desires to join the throngs of the missing. It is Bootie who does what no one even dares to conceive, namely, to embrace the resulting deaths of 9/11 not for any notion of grief or mourning but for personal gain: "He had been given—his fate—the precious opportunity to *be* again, not to be as he had been. Because as far as anyone knew, he *wasn't*."[23] Bootie changes his name to Ulrich New while his family holds a burial ceremony for him in Watertown, New York. The irony behind the live dead Bootie decentralizes, or *deterritorializes*, part of the grief discourse performed by the Thwaite clan in *The Emperor's Children*. By using 9/11 to create a new persona, it is almost as if Bootie can eschew the trauma narrative of his family and generate a different political territory for himself while everyone else keeps to their bourgeois liberalism.

Bootie's situation recalls Amis's statement about terrorists, "for whom death is not death—and for whom life is not life, either."²⁴ This is not to say that Bootie is a terrorist or even behaves like one, but rather that his actions shift the definition of death. The irony of the situation also plays a joke on the reader, who has been grieving Bootie's disappearance with the family throughout chapters 60 and 61 before he reappears in chapter 62.

The other ironic situation in the novel is also directly related to Bootie's disappearance, which the family deems a certain death. Murray is addressed frequently as a public intellectual and is asked about his feelings regarding his nephew. He states, "It's an indescribable loss. And ours is just one of thousands." As the public intellectual, Murray seems almost to address the reader as well; his voice in the novel tries to organize 9/11 for the curious reader who is also trying to make sense of it or at least understand its ramifications. The narrator elaborates on Murray's previous statement, commenting "and Murray couldn't help but be aware of the irony that Bootie's death had granted him greater nobility, and importance—he knew it to be false—as a man of justice, unswayed by the arrows of misfortune."²⁵ The irony here lies in the ways in which this death in the family authorizes Murray to oscillate between the private and public spheres. He can perform his speech acts with intellectual authority and as a New Yorker because he has been intimately affected by 9/11. Death becomes a privilege for him because he is grieving and negotiating post-9/11 trauma.

The final twist takes place in South Beach, Florida, instead of New York City, generating a geographic distance from the epicenter of the events. Danielle, after a failed suicide attempt, takes a trip with her mother, and they discuss Danielle's possible return to New York—"She had a film about liposuction to make. It seemed, in some lights, trivial, but it wasn't really. By the time it was finished, people would be tired of greater tragedies, and would be ready to watch it again." The humor here is for the reader: after 9/11, the liposuction must go on. Again, *The Emperor's Children* finds a way to make Danielle's life in New York more about the private sphere than about anything related to the public sphere or the collective history unfolding in the city. "People would be tired of greater tragedies," predicts Danielle in November 2001, in a novel published in 2006. In a way, this metafictional moment questions the novel's own place in a post-9/11 literary world, asking whether the "greater tragedy" of 9/11 has given way to other interests, or whether those interests—whatever they may be, but presented here as metaphorical contagion of ideological apparatuses—had been in place before 9/11 and afterward. That question of timing—of whether it is too soon to be inane rather than serious, personal instead of collective, or comedic, ironic, or satirical instead of tragic—marks the very last pages of the novel. Danielle runs into Bootie/Ulrich at the hotel where she is staying and where he now works. He explains to her the reason behind taking advantage of the disastrous events of 9/11: "I needed to go. I would be dead, otherwise. I needed—I haven't done anything wrong. If I would've killed myself otherwise, then I'd be dead, really dead. Maybe that would be better. Then would you be satisfied?"[26] The question of timing and the circumstances presented in the previous passage underline the final irony behind Bootie's disappearance. Bootie is still performing his first-person narrative in this dialogue, but he does so from a decentralized political position; he questions which deaths are worth more, which lives are *grievable* and *ungrievable*, to echo Butler's questions and categories.[27] Even though a metaphoric contagion of ideologies pervades the text, as expressed mostly through the bourgeois liberalism of the Thwaite family, the one character who refuses to make a pact with such contagion, Bootie, ends up becoming one of the missing in order to avoid the aforementioned ideological apparatus. That is, Bootie's decision to become part of the disappeared and carry the weight of the narrative's irony with him allows him to avoid the bourgeois entrapments of the emperor and his children.

The end of the novel puts the reader in a different kind of precarious position. The questions put to the characters, the systems of belief that are somewhat scrutinized by the children of the emperor, are also generated by and for the post-9/11 reader. The uses of irony within the context of the bourgeois liberalism of the text become a vital mechanism for creating a point of entry into post-9/11 politics and culture.

The Believers and the Question of Social Justice

Zoë Heller's 2009 novel *The Believers* also exhibits a very similar conta-gion of bourgeois, left-wing politics; all the main characters are actively engaged with the benefits and perils of being socially liberal and eco-nomically privileged. This section explores the socioeconomic complexi-ties of class in *The Believers* but also pays close attention to the use of irony as a narrative mechanism for perhaps questioning the intricacies of the metaphoric contagion of ideas and ideals.

The Believers takes place in an almost entirely post-9/11 world but opens by introducing the main character, Joel Litvinoff, meeting his future wife, Audrey, at a 1962 party while on his first trip to London. Joel goes on to describe his job to Audrey and explains that he works with disenfranchised people in the American South. He later elaborates: "'Negroes are the most disenfranchised people in America,' he said, 'and they're up against the most powerful people in America: the white establishment.'" The novel's opening pages then trace Joel back to 1962 in order to provide some background to his job forty years later. In 2002, Joel is working as a defense lawyer for Mohammed Hassani, described in the novel as a member of an Arab American group who visited an Al Qaeda training camp in Afghanistan back in 1998. Joel's opens his remarks for the case of *United States of America v. Mohammed Hassani* with the following statement about terrorism and fear: "Sometimes, in our earnest desire to protect this great country of ours, we can and do make errors. Errors that threaten to undermine the very liberties we are trying to protect. I am here to tell you that the presence of Mohammed Hassani in this courtroom today is one such error."[28] These lines highlight the metaphor of a family, a community, and a nation that have come under attack and must be protected from terrorists.[29] Heller's text voices the post-9/11 notion of a Christian United States fighting against an extrem-ist notion of Islam, but Joel uses such discourse to explain that Hassani has *not* engaged in terrorism. By resorting to the binary that joins Islam with extremism, Joel accepts the metaphor of feared contagion instead of rejecting it. Such a binary is put in place in the novel to organize a post-9/11 United States, as Butler notes at the beginning of *Precarious Life*.[30] Joel embraces ideas of terrorism in order to speak from within them and defend Hassani.[31] The novel pushes this pact with terrorism forward through Audrey, Joel's wife, who insists that her husband should defend Hassani "on grounds of legitimate Arab rage." Audrey utters Butler's observation about the instant gratification that arises from such moralistic accusation while attacking other political viewpoints.[32]

Immediately after establishing Joel as Hassani's lawyer, the novel introduces his socioeconomic position by anchoring it to his family home on Perry Street, next to houses that were renovated as the result of a certain "yuppie extravagance" on this "eighteenth-century street." The house on Perry Street is described not in architectural terms but rather in terms of a family history that is also imbued with privilege, as in the following description of the family tree and the family's adopted son, Lenny: "Joel had been very high on the idea of subverting traditional models of family life. Adopting seven-year-old Lenny was no mere act of bourgeois philanthropy, he had maintained, but a subversive gesture. . . . "[33] The novel parallels Joel's class with his notion of political subversion, and this is clearly picked up by the New York media.[34] Joel's character is introduced as a radical who has chosen to adopt un-American and terrorist ideas while living in the United States. In this first chapter, defending a terrorist means becoming one. Joel convinced Hassani not to make a deal with the prosecutor, in contrast with the other five men who were accused of terrorism and agreed to plea bargains. Hassani is the last man standing, trying, with Joel's defense, to prove that he is not a supporter of Al Qaeda, but Joel has to dive into the metaphoric uses of terrorism in order to defend his client.

At the end of the first chapter, Joel suffers a stroke as he is about to continue Hassani's defense. This moment halts not only his defense of Hassani but also his defense of terrorism. After Joel's stroke, Audrey is even more supportive of Hassani's defense and becomes another voice backing this seemingly willing contagion with terrorist ideas. Audrey talks to her friend Jean Himmelfarb about the ways in which Joel, almost as a terrorism-infected entity, has been "marginalized" and partly made the victim of "a bloody witch hunt going on in this country at the moment."[35] Both marginalization and witch hunts are used as mechanisms with which to present Joel in the novel and, more important, serve as a means of initially making him indistinguishable from Hassani.

This indistinctness between Joel and Hassani allows irony to play a crucial role in the lawyer-client relationship because both characters have to enter the realm of terrorism in order to explain that Hassani is *not* a terrorist. That is, Joel's initial portrait of Hassani as an "American citizen with three American children" is insufficient to defend him in a court of law in the United States. Instead, Joel has to explain the difference between terrorism and criticism of U.S. foreign policy in order to portray Hassani as an observer of the latter rather than the former. Irony becomes central to the novel, especially in relation to Hassani, because both terrorism and left-wing liberalism are presented as strict dogmas, as in Audrey's case: "For decades now, she had been dragging about the same unwieldy burden of a priori convictions, believing herself honor-bound to protect them against destruction at all costs. No new intelligence, no rational argument, could cause her to falter in her mission. Not even the cataclysmic events of the previous September had put her off stride for more than a couple of hours."[36] The more Audrey wants or claims to defend Hassani against the charges of terrorism, the more extremist her argument seems to be, as Jean notes. The novel, up to this point, weighs ideologies against each other, trying to find some common ground between the two. The end result is that it continues to highlight the ways in which both ideologies operate under very strict, almost unchangeable paradigms.

The novel proceeds with a flashback in order to delve further into a brief historiography of political movements, including the subject of terrorism. This comes forward in Karla's memory of something that happened when she was younger and living at home. The three Litvinoff children are sitting at the table with their father, discussing violent and nonviolent approaches to political mobilization, and Joel concludes, "If you look at history, you see that people who fight for their rights are often called terrorists, guerrillas, or whatever. But if they succeed—if they win their fight against oppression—they become national heroes. They become the new government."[37] The novel needs to go back in history, back in time, to a pre-9/11 world, in order to show that Joel had some kind of intellectual reflection on the subject before September 11, 2001.

The family's almost fanatic behavior, as seen in the words and actions of Audrey and Joel, is also narrated through Rosa, the Litvinoffs' younger daughter, who decides to study Orthodox Judaism after 9/11. Rosa, like her mother, engages with certain intellectual dogmas and demonstrates awareness of her intellectual trajectory: "For most of her life, she had been immunized against self-reproach by the certitudes of her socialist faith."[38] The past participle "immunized" allows the narrator to organize intellectual traditions through metaphors of contagion. Rosa had been *immunized* against guilt through socialism in her past, but "after a long and valiant battle against doubt, she had finally surrendered her political faith, and with it the densely woven screen of doctrinal abstraction through which she was accustomed to viewing the world." Rosa had clearly been working against what she considered "bourgeois liberalism," yet she realizes the irony behind her struggle: she wants to circumvent her socioeconomic privilege, but it is her bourgeois guilt as well as her privilege, to be without debt and with a college education, that allows her to work in an after-school program for a small salary. "She had become just another do-gooder, hoping to make a difference by taking underprivileged girls on museum trips."[39] Rosa proceeds in her intellectual struggle and one day is inexplicably moved while visiting a synagogue on Amsterdam Avenue.[40]

Her mother resorts to sarcasm to describe Rosa—"still dancing off the hora"—as well as ridicule: "Rosa's not *depressed*. She only went to Cuba to show everyone how special and interesting she was."[41] There are two crucial issues at stake here: first, Rosa's changing focus, from Cuban socialism to Orthodox Judaism; second, Audrey's perception of Rosa's performance of such interests, from "playing peasant" to "becoming Queen of the Matzoh." Besides deriding her daughter's religious interests, furthermore, Audrey then scoffs at the concept of religion, "it's all about repressing your sexual drives," a criticism then amplified through Hannah, Joel's mother, who also participates in the disapproval of Judaism.[42] *The Believers* places Judaism under more direct scrutiny than Islam, mostly because it comes from characters with family ties to the former and its traditions: "[Hannah's mother] took off her head-scarf and threw it in the water! . . . And why did she do this? So that her children and her children's children would not have to grow up under the tyranny of religion as she did. What do you think she would say today, if she could see her great-granddaughter futzing around with all the hocus-pocus and pie-in-the-sky that she rejected a century ago?"[43] Rosa finds herself at the crux of several critical remarks, including additional scrutiny from the Orthodox Jews themselves, who criticize her work instead of the religion. This takes place when she attends a Shabbaton, an extended Sabbath, in upstate New York and meets Rabbi Reinman's father-in-law, Mr. Riskin. The man admonishes her, saying that she should be working with her "own community" rather than providing after-school activities for African American girls in Harlem as she currently does. She responds that "these girls *are* my community" and adds that "they're New Yorkers just like I am."[44] Rosa's constant search for a community, for a center or a territory, be it in socialism or Judaism, underlines her partly decentralized or *deterritorialized* position, but as the novel progresses and she aligns herself more and more with Judaist principles, she ends up, quite ironically, in an ideological paradigm similar to the bourgeois liberalism she condemns.

In the novel, another means of immunization is being part of the bourgeoisie, as if its members are somehow protected from contagion from other socioeconomic groups. Audrey, for example, accomplishes this through her marriage to Joel, but after discovering that Joel had a three-year affair that resulted in a four-year-old child ("The great man of the Left having a secret bastard son," as she describes the situation), she immediately proceeds to try breaking her implicit agreement with her status as a left-wing bourgeois woman.[45] She starts by throwing some glasses to the floor in the kitchen and then goes on to break champagne glasses stolen from the Plaza Hotel as well as a Murano goblet.[46] The destruction of the glasses in the kitchen cabinets ends the second part of the novel and completes the somewhat metaphoric destruction of the Litvinoff family.

This metaphoric rupture with notions of class also comes by means of Rosa, who remains unsure about converting to Judaism after six months of study. She witnesses a mother hitting one of the girls from the after-school program and concludes, "'We're just one little program. Maybe we keep them off drugs for a while, and maybe we defer pregnancy for a few years, but they still have shitty parents and they still go to shitty schools and they're still going to end up with shitty jobs, or no jobs. Their'—she made an expansive gesture with her arms—'their class destiny is still going to be the same.'" "Bourgeois liberalism," as Rosa described it earlier, offers her students in the GirlPower program the socioeconomic resources they may not be able to access on their own. While Audrey tries to break her daughter's bourgeois, liberal bubble, Rosa becomes more aware of her place in it and the exclusion of others from it.

Capitalism does not emerge exempt from criticism, even from its able participants. A dinner party at the Litvinoff household while Joel is still in a coma becomes a heated family discussion, which is almost expected of all its participants. Tanya, Lenny's girlfriend, tries to defuse the tension by describing a launching party for a new Doritos chip, which suddenly becomes a concert by Enrique Iglesias, the pop music star. Mike, Karla's husband, interrupts Tanya's inane description of chips and ice sculptures by interjecting, "that's capitalism for you. Worshipping graven images of potato chips, while Kandahar burns."[47] In *The Believers*, especially as shown by this congregation of the family, except for Joel, no one is content with the ideological, political, or religious pacts the others have made. Capitalism, Liberalism, Conservatism, Judaism, Socialism, and Leftism are among the ideologies embraced by different members of the Litvinoff clan. And the stronger the self-deprecating humor in Heller's text, the more the text is able to get away with, in terms of those ideas from which it is distancing itself and, most important, those intellectual traditions with which the family members almost seem to be infected. The novel suggests that they do not see clearly, that all the *believers* in the novel want to believe in their respective ideologies.[48] In this case, to *believe* in capitalism is to want to be part of it, to be afflicted with all its symptoms.[49] The fascinating aspect of the novel is that it generates such belief in these ideas through the commitment of the believer and the derision of the nonbelievers. *The Believers* can be read as a novel of metaphoric contagion. The characters *believe* in intellectual traditions—of a political, cultural, and religious nature—and they want to be part of the traditions' contagion. Such infection is not to be feared, at least not for them.

The novel presents another example of metaphoric contagion through Karla, who is married but ends up flirting and eventually having sex with Khaled, an Egyptian man who owns the newspaper stand outside Columbia Presbyterian Hospital, where she works. They meet during a violent encounter, when one of the patients in Karla's ward attacks her and Khaled, who is in the hospital making a delivery, comes to her aid. Almost as expected, Khaled is initially introduced through Orientalist eyes, by a colleague of Karla's who cannot resist: "'*Arab*,' she mouthed silently."[50] *The Believers*, like *The Emperor's Children*, can muster criticism of Arabic or Islamic traditions, practices, or even terrorism only through these very minor characters.

The liberal Litvinoffs have another encounter with an ethnic/racial other, which in this case also works as a clear symbol of the family's socioeconomic status: a housekeeper who utters phrases such as "the visitors you was expecting." This use of the verb "to be" is tied to Mrs. Gates, the mother who slaps her own daughter at Rosa's after-school program with the accusation "You was smoking," as well as the girls in the program—"We wasn't slutty."[51] These minor moments in *The Believers* underline the education and socioeconomic class of the novel's marginal and marginalized characters, who in turn generate a contrast with the Litvinoff women.

Issues related to the Litvinoffs' bourgeois liberalism and its relation to race as well as ethnicity continue to be explored in *The Believers* when Karla goes to Ground Zero for a sexual encounter with Khaled in Battery Park City.[52] Karla had never been to Ground Zero before and was surprised by the fact that her hotel room faced that area. More importantly, she notices the cleaning up of the area. "The terrible piles of twisted metal that she had seen in newspaper photographs had been cleared away now," and "in their place lay an enormous, antiseptic gray scar."[53] The metaphoric scar refers generally to the metaphoric wound inflicted on September 11, but, more precisely, Karla's observation is about the reminder of the wound that had to be removed from the area. This point about Ground Zero goes hand in hand with the other ideas the characters commit to within the novel. For Karla, having sex with an Egyptian, presumably Muslim, according to the text, is her way of questioning her liberal and bourgeois upbringing. Rosa tries her version of socialism in Cuba and Judaism in New York, while Karla doubts marriage and her Republican husband by pursuing one of the objectionable others in her husband's binary, namely, a brown, Egyptian man.

The last chapters of *The Believers* intercalate several political events with discussions between members of the Litvinoff family. In its fourth and final part, the novel continues on to September 2, 2002, a moment in the text marked by Joel's ongoing coma, Audrey's reluctance to take him off the breathing machine ("Here it comes—the 'Let's Kill Joel' speech"), and, most relevant, Karla's ending of her six-week affair with Khaled while President Bush addresses a crowd at the Carpenters Joint Apprenticeship Center in Pittsburgh. The ending of Karla's and Khaled's affair is interwoven with some lines from Bush's speech on Labor Day:

"I'm sure your kids, they're wondering, why would you hate America. We didn't do anything to anybody. Well, they hate America because we love freedom. We cherish our freedoms. We value our freedoms."[54] The private sphere of Karla's life unfolds simultaneously with the rest of the United States' collective.

This same blurriness between the personal and collective aspects of the Litvinoff family also comes about in the antepenultimate chapter of the novel. From the Bush pro-war speech in September, the novel proceeds to the other end of the spectrum with actress Susan Sarandon addressing antiwar protesters in Central Park in October. Jean and Audrey attend the rally along with twenty thousand other protesters, and the occasion is marked by their brief discussion of their picnic of seafood salad, a baguette, and pâté—that is, the novel makes a political turn by presenting President Bush and his critics but does so by pairing the pro-war and antiwar speeches with a discussion of what is presented as a bourgeois outing. The political side of the moment is shadowed by the banality of the picnic. Furthermore, the text's narration of war politics is mixed with a minor discussion on race as Jean steps away from Audrey and runs into Rosa, who is chaperoning a group of girls from the afterschool program. "Jean smiled with the special goodwill that middle-aged white liberals reserve for young people of color." The novel then brings another of its ideological questions to the forefront by having Audrey and Rosa discuss the latter's interest in going to a yeshiva in Jerusalem. Audrey asks, "Why Judaism? That's what I want to know. Why did you have to choose the most reactionary religion?"[55] It is Audrey who turns shaming and extreme mockery—criticized by Butler, for example, as conservative and right-wing mechanisms—into tactics to be used against her daughter. The bourgeois liberals in the novel are unwilling to accept a discourse that is not theirs. The irony in Audrey is that she embodies the intolerance that she readily criticizes. The more she indulges in sarcasm, the more ironic her situation becomes. Unaware of her own bourgeois extremism, Audrey is not the end of irony but a manifestation of the irony that marked some post-9/11 criticism.

Furthermore, Joel's passing in the novel initially seems to represent the end of an era, but Audrey immediately creates out of his death the Litvinoff Foundation, which "will build on Joel's legacy by giving grants to progressive political and community initiatives that further the cause of social justice."[56] The memorial concludes with Audrey leading the attendees in a rendition of "The Internationale," bringing together her bourgeois liberal foundation and the anthem for international socialism. The metaphoric contagion of Audrey's ideology takes over the final moments of the novel; everyone happily agrees with her decision to put her position among the liberal bourgeoisie at the very center.

But this metaphoric contagion does not find a definite, final boundary in the novel's last pages. As *The Believers* further pushes the dichotomies influenced by the contagion of bourgeois liberalism, its final straw comes via Audrey's encounter with and acceptance of Joel's mistress, Berenice, and Berenice's son. In an almost predictable fashion, since the novel introduces Joel's interest in the American "disenfranchised" in its first pages, Berenice is a photographer who is also African American. At the memorial, Audrey not only announces the foundation but also welcomes Berenice into the Litvinoff family. Her clearly insincere kindness is the final sphere that the metaphoric contagion takes over. Audrey, as the new matriarch of the Litvinoff family, carries forward the family's bourgeois liberalism and will continue to "further the cause of social justice."

Grieving and Irony

Resolution in *The Emperor's Children* and *The Believers* depends on these two *grievable* deaths—those of Bootie and Joel—the opposite of Butler's "ungrievable deaths." These two deaths are partly necessary to the continuation of the novels' nation-building processes, or the imagined national community proposed by Benedict Anderson.[57] The United States, or the bourgeois liberal United States that counters Bush's post-9/11 United States, stands stronger at the end of both novels because the characters have endured death and its subsequent grief. It is also important to notice that these grievable deaths are marked with racial or ethnic privilege. *The Emperor's Children* clearly overlooks the racial or even ethnic dimension of its characters, and it could be argued that the story takes place in a post-racial New York, where the Thwaite family could be black or mixed race, but their ideological problems, at least the ones discussed here, clearly are marked by their privilege of being white. The Litvinoffs are non-practicing Jews, which becomes a family issue when a rabbi visits

Joel in his deathbed, and the novel makes it evident that they also live under what seems like white privilege—that is, there is a clear privilege that allows for the Thwaite and Litvinoff families to finally accomplish some kind of closure after enduring a *grievable* death. But each family's grief is somehow subverted by additional, unexpected circumstances.

These circumstances, tied to the aftermath of 9/11, are central parts of both novels, but the causes or historical background of September 11, 2001, are not narrated or referenced in either one. In *The Emperor's* *Children*, the main concern is the effects of the events in the lives of the white, bourgeois characters. The text narrates pain, but no blame, no condemnation. Even Murray Thwaite, the public intellectual, takes the silent road. *The Believers* adopts a similar narrative standpoint: 9/11 is used as a superficial entry into social justice but ends up being a setup for the Litvinoff Foundation, after the liberal lawyer and patriarch dies. In both novels, the characters, in their complicit silence, are critical only of the government's post-9/11 violent excesses. These characters fear being infected with a Bush-era, right-wing, conservative ideology and therefore run toward the other metaphoric infection, namely, the "bourgeois liberalism" described by Rosa.

This narration of the effects of 9/11 is also tied to the fact that both *The Emperor's Children* and *The Believers* follow chronological time lines and, hence, sequential narratives. The two novels almost depend on chronology and structured order for generating their respective pacts with 9/11 as a series of narrative events that alter the plots and dramas of their characters' lives. September 11 works as a point in the plot—more than halfway through in *The Emperor's Children* and as a turning point in the recent past of the characters in *The Believers*. The way in which these characters work toward their notion of social justice based on an apparent loss of First Worldism after 9/11, in both their public and private realms, allows them to reinforce and underline their positions within an ideological apparatus while trying to insert themselves as active agents for change in debates about post-9/11 politics.

Of the two novels examined in this chapter, only *The Emperor's Children* narrates the events of 9/11 and their aftermath in present time, yet the text seems unable to speak about the collective national discourse that immediately followed. *The Emperor's Children* does not delve into the "hegemonic grammar,"[58] to borrow Butler's phrase, generated in the United States after 9/11. The text carefully avoids key binarisms that were reactivated on 9/11 and resists uttering the word "terrorism" and its related discourse. The same could almost be said for *The Believers* since the issue of terrorism deflates as quickly, when Joel suffers his stroke early in the novel. Once his brain is no longer working, any questions about terrorism are suddenly out of the scope of the novel because he is no longer defending Hassani.

If 9/11 brings forward questions about the precariousness of life, the Thwaite family believes that Bootie is the only one who has suffered from this state because of his disappearance; he is alive, however, and the novel almost laughs at the family's grief. Bootie in *The Emperor's Children* is perhaps the only character who is close to a partial decentralization of the first-person narrative that is never present in *The Believers*, or many other 9/11 novels for that matter. The novel achieves this decentralized or *deterritorialized* character in part because Bootie lacks a notion of home, unlike every other character studied here, but the process is never fully accomplished within the chronological form of Messud's novel.

These novels seek to explore the mechanisms—literary, historical, political—by which their characters try to avoid ideological traps that they deem unfair and unjust even as these characters refuse to take a critical approach to their almost default ideologies. The metaphorical and ideological contagion in *The Emperor's Children* and *The Believers* could also be related to the novels' setting in New York City; they are centralized narratives at the epicenter of the 9/11 events. It is almost as if the characters cannot see their ideological blind spots, or are unwilling to see them, because of their location; they cannot read and perceive the issues that are right under their noses.

Finally, this metaphoric contagion creates a certain resistance to the didactic and prescriptive tone in Butler's argument as well as in Gray's and Rothberg's criticism of post-9/11 literature. Bootie in *The Emperor's Children* and Audrey in *The Believers* may not be the exemplary characters that would perhaps fulfill the need for deterritorialized narratives, but both surely introduce a point of resistance and contradictions that may not necessarily work against the seriousness of post-9/11 aesthetics and politics. These two characters—one who uses his disappearance as a way out of the epitome of a bourgeois liberal family and the other who embodies a certain bourgeois liberal hypocrisy—resist the heavy

ALBERTO S. GALINDO

solemnity that characterized a post-9/11 world, defying as well the way in which other characters perceive them. Bootie and Audrey are not read by other characters as people who would resolve their respective plots as they do. This is the final irony ciphered in these novels. The other characters, those who *read* the lives of Bootie and Audrey, fall victim to the metaphoric contagion of bourgeois liberalism but are not necessarily infected or affected by irony. This irony, or ironic way of reading against the gravity of 9/11, is available only to Danielle in *The Emperor's Children* and simply is alluded to in Audrey's self-perception in *The Believers*. Perhaps the ultimate challenge rises from the pages of these novels to their readers, who may end up prey to irony's metaphoric contagion.

NOTES

1   Judith Butler, *Precarious Life* (London: Verso, 2004), 1.

2   Zoë Heller, *The Believers* (New York: HarperCollins, 2009), 59.

3   For a study of metaphors of contagion as they relate to Communism, see Priscilla Wald, "Viral Cultures: Microbes and Politics in the Cold War," in *Contagious: Cultures, Carriers, and the Outbreak Narrative* (Durham, N.C.: Duke University Press, 2008).

4   Kristiaan Versluys, *Out of the Blue: September 11 and the Novel* (New York: Columbia University Press, 2009), 183.

5   The connection between the style of *The Emperor's Children* and *The Believers* has been noted before, as in the case of Jill Abramson's review of the latter: "There are familiar overtones in *The Believers*. Its depiction of a family galaxy that spins around an accomplished, famous and amorous father is reminiscent of Claire Messud's satirical novel *The Emperor's Children*" (Jill Abramson, "The Tribe of Joel," *New York Times*, March 6, 2009). Fatema Ahmed makes a similar comparison in her review of *The Believers* for *New Statesman* (September 25, 2008) as does Joanna Briscoe in her review of the same novel for the *Guardian* (September 20, 2008).

6   Heller, *The Believers*, 26. Gramsci's quote is an indirect reference to Romain Rolland. Translations of Gramsci's text from his letter of December 19, 1929, vary; consider the following variation on the subjects of the sentences in contrast with the quote from Heller's text: "My own state of mind synthesizes these two feelings and transcends them: my mind is pessimistic, but my will is optimistic" (Antonio Gramsci, *Letters from Prison*, trans. Lynne Lawner [New York: Harper Colophon, 1975], 159). Gramsci quotes Rolland directly in an unsigned piece from 1920 for the weekly

L'Ordine Nuovo: "The socialist conception of the revolutionary process is characterized by two fundamental features that Romain Rolland has summed up in his watchword: 'pessimism of the intellect, optimism of the will.'" Antonio Gramsci, *Selections from Political Writings, 1910–1920*, trans. John Matthews (New York: International Publishers, 1977), 188.

7   Wald traces the genealogy of the concept of social contagion back to Robert Ezra Park while relating it to Sigmund Freud and Émile Durkheim as well: "the term *contagion* suggested a connective and transformative force and was commonly used to describe how an individual got caught up in the spirit and actions of a group, surrendering personal agency and even rational thought to the collective will." Furthermore, she discusses social contagion and the ways in which "ideas and attitudes spread like germs because of individual proximity and interdependence." Wald, *Contagious*, 131, 137.

8   Chantal Mouffe explores Gramsci's concept of ideology and its relation to intellectuals: "They [the intellectuals] are the ones in charge of elaborating and spreading organic ideologies, and they are the ones who will have to realize moral and intellectual reform" (Chantal Mouffe, "Hegemony and Ideology in Gramsci," in *Gramsci and Marxist Theory* [London: Routledge and Kegan Paul, 1979], 187).

9   Martin Amis, *The Second Plane* (New York: Alfred A. Knopf, 2008), ix.

10   Trauma theory has been invoked as starting point in various articles and books. Versluys traces many of the uses of trauma in the introduction, "9/11: The Discursive Responses," to his *Out of the Blue*.

11   Gray turns to Freud and Cathy Caruth in order to study some trauma-related issues at stake in novels such as Don DeLillo's *Falling Man* (2007), Ken Kalfus's *A Disorder Peculiar to the Country* (2006), Messud's *The Emperor's Children* (2006), and John Updike's *Terrorist* (2006). Richard Gray, "Open Doors, Closed Minds: American Prose Writing at a Time of Crisis," *American Literary History* 21, no. 1 (2009): 128–48.

12   Michael Rothberg, "A Failure of the Imagination: Diagnosing the Post-9/11 Novel: A Response to Richard Gray," *American Literary History* 21, no. 1 (2009): 152–58.

13   Gilles Deleuze and Félix Guattari, *Kafka: Toward a Minor Literature* (Minneapolis: University of Minnesota Press, 1986).

14   For Danielle, the events on that day seemed "all too big and too much to take in and she wanted, now, to turn it off, just to turn it all off—and then she kicked off her shoes and with her skirt rucked up, climbed back into her beautiful bed and pulled the duvet—such soft cotton, so very fine, Murray's special sheets, and they smelled of him—over her head, as she used to do as a child, and she thought that she should cry, she thought

that perhaps later she might cry" (Claire Messud, *The Emperor's Children* [New York: Alfred A. Knopf, 2006], 373).

15 Ibid., 373.

16 Ibid., 375, 376. The exaggeration of Ludovic's statement reads as follows: "This is necrophiliac pornography. . . . But what good does it do to pretend they'll all come home, that they're just wandering around Manhattan in a post-traumatic daze?" Ibid., 376.

17 Ibid., 383.

18 Butler, *Precarious Life*, 7.

19 Transcript of President Bush's address to a joint session of Congress on September 20, 2001, http://archives.cnn.com/2001/US/09/20/gen. bush.transcript/.

20 William R. Jones studies these kinds of statements in "'People Have to Watch What They Say': What Horace, Juvenal, and 9/11 Can Tell Us about Satire and History," *Helios* 36, no. 1 (2009): 27–53. Meghan O'Rourke poses the same question in her review of *The Emperor's Children*, "The End of Irony," *New York Times*, August 27, 2006.

21 Amis, *The Second Plane*, 85–86.

22 "He'd chosen Miami because when the station opened at five, it was the farthest and earliest one could go." Messud, *The Emperor's Children*, 395. Bootie's destination brings to mind President Bush's remarks to the nation from Chicago's O'Hare International Airport: "Get on board; do your business around the country; fly and enjoy America's great destination spots; get down to Disney World in Florida." George W. Bush, "Remarks to Airline Employees in Chicago, Illinois," September 27, 2001, http://www.presidency.ucsb.edu/ws/index.php?pid=65084.

23 Messud, *The Emperor's Children*, 393.

24 Amis, *The Second Plane*, 22.

25 Messud, *The Emperor's Children*, 414.

26 Ibid., 425, 429.

27 Butler, *Precarious Life*, 20.

28 Heller, *The Believers*, 11, 22.

29 Joel elaborates furthermore, "You have been told that Mohammed Hassani is a supporter of terrorism. You have been told that he hates America and wants to aid and abet those who would destroy it." Ibid., 22.

30 Butler draws the beginnings of these post-9/11 binarisms from Bush's "Either you're with us or you're with the terrorists." She mentions other long-standing political and cultural binaries, such as the East-West divide and civilization versus barbarism (Butler, *Precarious Life*, 2).

31 Joel continues, "Does he possess strong religious beliefs? Yes. But remember, ladies and gentlemen, whatever the prosecution tries to

suggest, it is not Islam that is on trial in this courtroom." Heller, *The Believers*, 22.

32   Ibid., 23, 16.

33   Ibid., 26. Joel's notion of political and economic subversion even affects his perception of Lenny: "had Lenny ever put his rebellious impulses to some principled use: run away to join the Sandinistas, say, or vandalized U.S. Army recruiting offices" (ibid).

34   Consider, for example, the way in which Joel's defense of Hassani draws the attention of the press, including the *New York Post*, which describes him as a "rent-a-radical with a long history of un-Americanism" (ibid., 28).

35   Ibid., 35.

36   Ibid., 22, 37.

37   Ibid., 80.

38   Ibid., 58.

39   Ibid., 59.

40   Rosa was "filled with a mysterious, euphoric sense of belonging" (ibid., 61).

41   Ibid., 37, 38.

42   Ibid., 38.

43   Ibid., 93–94.

44   Ibid., 116.

45   Ibid., 184.

46   Ibid., 160.

47   Ibid., 216.

48   Amis discusses the frequent use of the verb "to believe" as part of the "re-emergence of sentiment as the prince of the critical utensils" (Amis, *The Second Plane*, 18).

49   This paradigm of belief can be contrasted with Amis's fictional description of Muhammad Atta, one of hijackers on the first plane to hit the World Trade Center: "You *needed* the belief system, the ideology, the ardor. You had to have it. The core reason was good enough for the mind. But it couldn't carry the body" (Heller, *The Believers*, 116).

50   Ibid., 132. Consider a similar example from *The Emperor's Children*, in which Judy's hairdresser, who styles her hair the afternoon of September 11, describes the whole set of events as "'awful. It's those Arabs,' she said, pronouncing it *Ay-rabs*" (Messud, *The Emperor's Children*, 379).

51   Heller, *The Believers*, 170, 193.

52   Joel's sister-in-law, Julie, is the first to mention Ground Zero in *The Believers* when she visits Joel and Audrey in New York. As she is about to leave to visit Ground Zero with her husband, Colin, she asks Joel for a place "anywhere down there that you'd recommend for lunch," but Joel decides not to answer her question. As a tourist from England, Julie clearly speaks

from her standpoint of privilege. Her question emphasizes Ground Zero as a tourist destination (ibid., 24).

53 Ibid., 253.

54 Ibid., 283, 288.

55 Ibid., 311, 313.

56 Ibid., 330.

57 Wald analyzes the ways in which Anderson's *Imagined Communities* presents a useful concept for relating a strong sense of national belonging to reaction to the fear of an outbreak. Wald, *Contagious*, 51–53.

58 Butler, *Precarious Life*, 13.

BIBLIOGRAPHY

Adams, Tim. "The Library in the Body." Review of *The Body Artist*, by Don DeLillo. *Observer*, February 11, 2001. http://www.guardian.co.uk/books/2001/feb/11/fiction.dondelillo.

Agamben, Giorgio. "Security and Terror." Translated by Carolin Emcke. *Theory & Event* 5, no. 4 (2001).

————. *The Open: Man and Animal*. Translated by Kevin Attell. Stanford, Calif.: Stanford University Press, 2002.

————. *State of Exception*. Translated by Kevin Attell. Chicago: University of Chicago Press, 2005.

Aisenberg, Andrew Robert. *Contagion: Disease, Government, and the "Social Question" in Nineteenth-Century France*. Stanford, Calif.: Stanford University Press, 1999.

"Al Qaeda's New Front." *Frontline*, October 12, 2004. PBS. http:www.pbs.org/wgbh/pages/frontline/shows/front/map/bruguiere.html.

Allen, Franklin, and Douglas Gale. "Financial Contagion." *Journal of Political Economy* 108, no. 1 (2000): 1–33.

Alvarez, Lizette. "Britain's Mainstream Muslims Find Voice." *New York Times*, March 6, 2005.

Amis, Martin. *The Second Plane*. New York: Alfred A. Knopf, 2008.

Anderson, Warwick. "Natural Histories of Infectious Disease: Ecological Vision in Twentieth-Century Bioscience." *Osiris* 19 (2004): 39–61.

Andresen, Margot. "Avian Flu: WHO Prepares for the Worst." *Canadian Medical Journal* 170, no. 5 (March 2004): 777.

Anonymous. *Through Our Enemies' Eyes: Osama Bin Laden, Radical Islam, and the Future of America.* Washington, D.C.: Brassey's, 2002.

Ashley, Richard. "Living on the Borderlines: Man, Poststructuralism and War." In *International/Intertextual Relations,* edited by James Der Derian and Michael Shapiro, 259–321. Lexington, MA: Lexington Books, 1989.

Ashraf, Haroon. "David Heymann—WHO's Public Health Guru." *Lancet Infectious Diseases* 4, no. 12 (2004): 785–88.

Bai, Matt. "The Framing Wars." *New York Times Magazine,* July 12, 2005.

Bashford, Alison. "Global Biopolitics and the History of World Health." *History of the Human Sciences* 19, no. 1 (2006): 67–88.

Baudrillard, Jean. *America.* Translated by Chris Turner. London: Verso, 1996.

———. *Cool Memories.* Translated by Chris Turner. London: Verso, 1990.

———. *Cool Memories II: 1987–1990.* Translated by Chris Turner. Durham, N.C.: Duke University Press, 1996.

———. *Fragments: Cool Memories III, 1991–1995.* Translated by Emily Agar. London: Verso, 1997.

———. *L'autre par lui-même: Habilitation.* Paris: Galilée, 1987.

———. *Paroxysm: Interviews with Philippe Petit.* Translated by Chris Turner. London: Verso, 1998.

———. *The Perfect Crime.* Translated by Chris Turner. London: Verso, 1996.

———. *The Vital Illusion.* Edited by Julia Witwer. New York: Columbia University Press, 2000.

Becker, Karen. "Avian and Influenza Pandemics: A Threat to the Asia-Pacific Community." Submitted to APEC Meeting on Avian and Pandemic Influenza Preparedness and Response, Brisbane, Australia 31 October–1 November 2005, available at http://unpan1.un.org/intradoc/groups/public/documents/apcity/unpan022560.pdf.

Belford, Aubrey. "Indonesia's Bird Flu Warrior Takes on the World." Agence France-Presse, October 12, 2008.

Benjamin, Walter. "Thesis on the Philosophy of History." In *Illuminations: Essays and Reflections,* edited and with an introduction by Hannah Arendt, 253–64. Translated by Harry Zohn. New York: Schocken Books, 1968.

———. "The Work of Art in the Age of Mechanical Reproduction." In *Illuminations: Essays and Reflections,* edited and with an introduction by Hannah Arendt. Translated by Harry Zohn, 217–51. New York: Schocken Books, 1968.

Bettancourt, Luis M. A., Arial Cintron-Arias, David I. Kaiser, and Carlos Castillo-

Chavez. "The Power of a Good Idea: Quantitative Models." Santa Fe Institute Working Paper, February 6. Santa Fe, N.Mex.: Santa Fe Institute, 2005.

Bhat, Amar. "Remarks by the APEC Health Task Force Chair." http://www. apec.org/apec/documents_reports/health_task_force/2005.html#AI.

Blanchard, Christopher M. *Al Qaeda: Statements and Evolving Ideology.* CRS Report for Congress, February 4, 2005. Washington, D.C.: U.S. Department of State, 2005.

Bleiker, Roland. "Art after 9/11." *Alternatives: Global, Local, Political* 31, no. 1 (2006): 77–99.

Bloom, Mia. *Dying to Kill: The Allure of Suicide Terror.* New York: Columbia University Press, 2005.

Borradori, Giovanna. *Philosophy in a Time of Terror: Dialogues with Jürgen Habermas and Jacques Derrida.* Chicago: University of Chicago Press, 2004.

Bradsher, Keith. "Global Effort Attracts $1.9 Billion in Pledges to Battle Bird Flu." *New York Times,* January 19, 2006.

Brandon, James. "Koranic Duel Eases Terror." *Christian Science Monitor,* February 4, 2005.

Brown, Theodore M., Marcos Cueto, and Elizabeth Fee. "The World Health Organization and the Transition from 'International' to 'Global' Health." *American Journal of Public Health* 96, no. 1 (2006): 622–72.

Butler, Judith. *Gender Trouble: Feminism and the Subversion of Identity.* New York: Routledge, 1999.

———. *Precarious Life.* London: Verso, 2004.

Calain, Philippe. "From the Field Side of the Binoculars: A Different View on Global Public Health Surveillance." *Health Policy and Planning* 22, no. 1 (2007): 13–20.

Caldwell, Anne. "Bio-sovereignty and the Emergence of Humanity." *Theory & Event* 7, no. 2 (2004).

Campbell, David. *Writing Security: United States Foreign Policy and the Politics of Identity.* Minneapolis: University of Minnesota Press, 1998.

Campbell, Timothy. "Bios, Immunity, Life: The Thought of Roberto Esposito." *Diacritics* 36, no. 2 (2006): 6–11.

Canadian Broadcasting Corportation. "The Next Pandemic?" http://www.cbc. ca/news/background/avianflu.

Chambers, Whittaker. "I Was the Witness." *Saturday Evening Post,* February 23, 1952, 22–23, 48–63.

Chaon, Anne. "France Joins Europe Flu Vaccine Sell-Off." Agence France-Presse, January, 3, 2010.

Christian, Michael D. "Development of a Triage Protocol for Critical Care during an Influenza Pandemic." *Canadian Medical Association* 175, no. 11 (2006): 1377–81. http://www.cmaj.ca/cgi/eletters/175/11/1377.

177

Clausewitz, Carl von. *On War*. Oxford: Oxford University Press, 2007.

Cohen, Deborah, and Philip Carter. "WHO and the Pandemic Flu 'Conspiracies.'" *British Medical Journal* 340 (June 12, 2010): 1274–79.

Coleman, William. *Death Is a Social Disease: Public Health and Political Economy in Early Industrial France*. Madison: University of Wisconsin Press, 1982.

Collier, Stephen J., and Andrew Lakoff. "The Problem of Securing Health." In *Biosecurity Interventions: Global Health and Security in Question*, edited by Stephen J. Collier and Andrew Lakoff, 7–32. New York: Columbia University Press, 2008.

Culliton, Barbara. "Emerging Viruses, Emerging Threat." *Science* 247, no. 4940 (January 19, 1990): 279–80.

Cuthbertson, Ian. "Prisons and the Education of Terrorists." *World Policy Journal* 21, no. 3 (Fall 2004): 15–22.

Dalby, Simon. "Reading Kaplan's 'Coming Anarchy.'" In *The Geopolitics Reader*, edited by Gearóid Ó Tuathail, Simon Dalby, and Paul Routledge, 197–203. London: Routledge, 1998.

Dallmayr, Fred. "An 'Inoperative' Global Community? Reflections on Nancy." In *On Jean-Luc Nancy: The Sense of Philosophy*, edited by Darren Sheppard, Simon Sparks, and Colin Thomas, 174–96. London: Routledge, 1997.

Davis, Mike. *The Monster at Our Door: The Global Threat of Avian Flu*. New York: The New Press, 2005.

Deleuze, Gilles, and Félix Guattari. *Kafka: Toward a Minor Literature*. Minneapolis: University of Minnesota Press, 1986.

DeLillo, Don. *The Body Artist*. New York: Scribner, 2001.

———. *Cosmopolis*. New York: Scribner, 2003.

———. *Great Jones Street*. Boston: Houghton Mifflin, 1973.

———. *The Names*. New York: Random House, 1989.

———. "'An Outsider in This Society': Interview with Don DeLillo." Interview by Anthony DeCurtis. *South Atlantic Quarterly* 89, no. 2 (1990), 281–304.

———. "The Power of History." *New York Times Magazine*, September 7, 1997. http://www.nytimes.com/library/books/090797article3.html.

———. *Underworld*. New York: Scribner, 1997.

Derrida, Jacques. "Faith and Knowledge: The Two Sources of 'Religion' at the Limits of Reason Alone." In *Acts of Religion: Jacques Derrida*, edited by Gil Anidjar, 40–101. New York: Routledge, 2002.

———. *Negotiations*. Edited and translated by Elizabeth Rottenberg. Stanford, Calif.: Stanford University Press, 2001.

———. *On Touching—Jean-Luc Nancy*. Translated by Christine Irizarry. Stanford, Calif.: Stanford University Press, 2005.

———. "Peine de mort et souveraineté." *Divinatio* 15 (2002): 13–38.

———. *Rogues: Two Essays on Reason*. Translated by Pascale-Anne Brault and Michael Naas. Stanford, Calif.: Stanford University Press, 2005.

Diamond, Jared. *Guns, Germs, and Steel: The Fates of Human Societies.* New York: W. W. Norton, 1997.

Donnelly, John. "Specialists Say TB Case a Sign of Things to Come." *Boston Globe,* June 4, 2007.

Doughton, Sandi. "Gates Foundation Launches 3rd Initiative in China." *Seattle Times,* March 31, 2009.

Drexler, Madeline. *Secret Agents: The Menace of Emerging Infections.* New York: Penguin Books, 2002.

Epstein, Joshua M. "Modeling Civil Violence: An Agent-Based Computational Approach." *Proceedings of the National Academy of Sciences* 99, suppl. no. 3 (May 14, 2003): 7243–50.

Esposito, Roberto. *Bios: Biopolitics and Philosophy.* Translated by Timothy Campbell. Minneapolis: University of Minnesota Press, 2008.

Ewald, François. "Insurance and Risk." In *The Foucault Effect: Studies in Governmentality,* edited by Graham Burchell, Colin Gordon, and Peter Miller, 197–210. Chicago: University of Chicago Press, 1991.

Farmer, Paul. *Infections and Inequalities: The Modern Plagues.* Berkeley: University of California Press, 2001.

Fatal Contact: Bird Flu in America. DVD. Directed by Richard Pearce. Culver City, Calif.: Sony Pictures Home Entertainment, 2006.

Fattah, Hassan M. "Jordan Is Preparing to Tone Down the Islamic Bombast in Textbooks." *New York Times,* June 12, 2005.

Fauci, Anthony. "Race against Time." *Nature* 435 (May 26, 2005): 423–24.

Fearnley, Lyle. "'From Chaos to Controlled Disorder': Syndromic Surveillance, Bioweapons, and the Pathological Future." *ARC Working Paper* no. 5 (2005). http://anthropos-lab.net/wp/publications/2007/08/workingpaper105.pdf.

Fee, Elizabeth, and Dorothy Porter. "Public Health, Preventive Medicine and Professionalization: England and America in the Nineteenth Century." In *Medicine in Society: Historical Essays,* edited by Andrew Wear, 249–75. Cambridge: Cambridge University Press, 1992.

Fernandez, Jorge. "Ebola Takes to the Road." In *Sovereign Lives: Power in Global Politics,* edited by Jenny Edkins, Michael J. Shapiro, and Véronique Pin-Fat, 189–210. London: Routledge, 2004.

Fidler, David P. "From International Sanitary Conventions to Global Health Security: The New International Health Regulations." *Chinese Journal of International Law* 4, no. 2 (2005): 325–92.

———. "Influenza Virus Samples, International Law, and Global Health Diplomacy." *Emerging Infectious Diseases* 14, no. 1 (2008): 88–94.

Fidler, David P., Howard Markel, and Lawrence O. Gostin. "Extensively Drug-Resistant Tuberculosis: An Isolation Order, Public Health Powers, and Global Crisis." *JAMA* 298, no. 1 (2007): 83–86.

Foucault, Michel. "The Birth of Biopolitics." In *Ethics, Subjectivity and Truth,* edited by Paul Rabinow, 73–79. Translated by Robert Hurley et al. Vol. 1 of *Essential Works of Foucault 1954–1984*. New York: New Press, 2000.

———. "Governmentality." In *Power*, edited by James D. Faubion, 201–22. Translated by Robert Hurley. Vol. 3 of *Essential Works of Foucault 1954–1984*. New York: New Press, 2000.

———. *The History of Sexuality, Volume 1*. Translated by Robert Hurley. New York: Vintage Books, 1978.

———. *The Order of Things*. London: Routledge, 1989.

———. *"Society Must Be Defended": Lectures at the Collège de France, 1975–1976*. Edited by Mauro Bertani and Alessandro Fontana. Translated by David Macey. New York: Pantheon, 2003.

Fouchier, Ron. "Global Task Force for Influenza." *Nature* 435 (May 26, 2005): 419–20.

Franklin, Sarah. "Stem Cells R Us: Emergent Life Forms and the Global Biological." In *Global Assemblages, Technology, Politics and Ethics as Anthropological Problems*, edited by Aihwa Ong and Stephen J. Collier, 59–78. London: Blackwell, 2005.

Fukuyama, Francis. *The End of History and the Last Man*. London: Penguin Books, 1992.

Fumento, Michael. "Fuss and Feathers: Pandemic Panic over the Avian Flu." *Weekly Standard*, November 21, 2005.

Garrett, Laurie. *The Coming Plague: Newly Emerging Diseases in a World Out of Balance*. New York: Farrar, Straus and Giroux, 1994.

———. "The Next Pandemic?" *Foreign Affairs*, July–August 2005: 3–23

Gerstman, Burt B. *Epidemiology Kept Simple: An Introduction to Traditional and Modern Epidemiology*. Hoboken, N.J.: Wiley Liss, 2003.

Giddens, Anthony. *The Consequences of Modernity*. Stanford, Calif.: Stanford University Press, 1990.

Gladwell, Malcolm. *The Tipping Point: How Little Things Can Make a Big Difference*. Boston: First Back Bay, 2002.

Glassner, Barry. *The Culture of Fear*. New York: Basic Books, 1999.

Gompf, Sandra G., Jordan Lewis, Eknath Naik, and Kaley Tash. "The Infectious Disease Physician and Microbial Bioterrorism." In *Microorganisms and Bioterrorism*, edited by Burt Anderson, Herman Friedman, and Mauro Bendinelli, 31–38. New York: Springer Science and Business Media, 2006.

Gordis, Leon. *Epidemiology*. 3rd ed. Philadelphia: Elsevier Saunders, 2004.

Gramsci, Antonio. *Letters from Prison*. Translated by Lynne Lawner. New York: Harper Colophon, 1975.

———. *Selections from Political Writings, 1910–1920*. Translated by John Matthews. New York: International Publishers, 1977.

Gray, Richard. "Open Doors, Closed Minds: American Prose Writing at a Time of Crisis." *American Literary History* 21, no. 1 (2009): 128–48.

Haass, Richard N. Speech to the Council on Foreign Relations, New York, October 15, 2001.

Hardt, Michael, and Antonio Negri. *Empire*. Cambridge, Mass.: Harvard University Press, 2000.

————. *Multitude: War and Democracy in the Age of Empire*. New York: Penguin, 2004.

Heller, Zoë. *The Believers*. New York: HarperCollins, 2009.

Henderson, D. A. *Smallpox: The Death of a Disease*. New York: Prometheus, 2009.

Henderson, D. H. "Surveillance Systems and Intergovernmental Cooperation." In *Emerging Viruses*, edited by Stephen S. Morse, 283–89. New York: Oxford University Press, 1993.

Heymann, David. "The International Response to the Outbreak of SARS in 2003." *Philosophical Transactions of the Royal Society of London B*, 359 (2004): 1127–29.

Hill, Alison L., David G. Rand, Martin A. Nowak, and Nicholas A. Christakis. "Infectious Disease Modeling of Social Contagion in Networks." *PLoS Computational Biology* 6, no. 11 (2010): 1–15.

Hines, William. "The AIDS Epidemic: A Report from the Front Lines." *Washington Post*, October 11, 1987.

Hoffman, Bruce. "Unconventional Threats and Capabilities." Testimony to the House Armed Services Committee, Subcommittee on Terrorism, Unconventional Threats and Capabilities, 109th Cong., 2nd sess., February 16, 2006.

Hogan, Chuck. *The Blood Artists*. New York: Avon Books, 1998.

Hooker, Claire. "Drawing the Lines: Danger and Risk in the Age of SARS." In *Medicine at the Border: Disease, Globalization, and Security, 1850 to the Present*, edited by Alison Bashford, 179–95. Houndsmill, Basingstoke, Hampshire, England, and New York: Palgrave Macmillan, 2007.

Hotel Rwanda. Directed by Terry George. DVD. Century City, Calif.: MGM, 2004.

House Committee on Homeland Security. *The 2007 XDR-TB Incident: A Breakdown at the Intersection of Homeland Security and Public Health*. 110th Cong., 1st sess., 2007.

"International Health Regulations: The Challenges Ahead." *Lancet* 369, no. 9575 (May 26, 2007): 1763.

Joint Chiefs of Staff. *Joint Vision 2020: America's Military; Preparing for Tomorrow*. Washington, D.C.: Government Printing Office, 2000. http://www.dtic.mil/doctrine/jel/jfq_pubs/1225.pdf.

Jones, William R. "'People Have to Watch What They Say': What Horace, Juvenal, and 9/11 Can Tell Us about Satire and History." *Helios* 36, no. 1 (2009): 27–53.

Kallen, Horace M. "Democracy vs. the Melting Pot." *Nation* 100 (February 18, 25, 1915): 190–94, 217–20.

181

Kaplan, David E. "Hearts, Minds, and Dollars." *U.S. News and World Report*, April 25, 2005.

Kaplan, Robert. "The Coming Anarchy." *Atlantic Monthly* 273, no. 2 (1994): 44–76.

———. "Supremacy by Stealth." *Atlantic Monthly* 292, no. 1 (July–August 2003): 66–83.

Kazatchkine, Veronique and Michael Martinache. "Swine Flu: Rich Nations' Spending Spurs Ethics Row." Agence France-Presse, August 1, 2009.

Kepel, Gilles. *The War for Muslim Minds.* Cambridge, Mass.: Harvard University Press, 2004.

Kilcullen, David J. "Countering Global Insurgency." *Journal of Strategic Studies* 28, no. 4 (August 2005): 597–617.

King, Nicholas. "Security, Disease, Commerce: Ideologies of Post-colonial Global Health." *Social Studies of Science* 32, no. 5–6 (2002): 763–89.

Kirby, Jason. "Europe Gets Greeced." *MacLean's*, May 17, 2010. http://www2.macleans.ca/2010/05/07/europe-gets-greeced/.

Knauer, Nancy J. "Homosexuality as Contagion: From the Well of Loneliness to the Boy Scouts." *Hofstra Law Review* 29, no. 2 (2000): 401–501.

Krause, Richard M. Foreword to *Emerging Viruses*, edited by Stephen S. Morse, xvii–xix. New York: Oxford University Press, 1993.

———. "The Origin of Plagues: Old and New." *Science* 257, no. 1 (August 21, 1992): 1073–77.

Kraut, Alan M. *Silent/Travelers: Germs, Genes, and the "Immigrant Menace."* Baltimore, Md.: Johns Hopkins University Press, 1994.

Langmuir, Alexander. "The Surveillance of Communicable Diseases of National Importance." *New England Journal of Medicine* 268, no. 4 (1963): 182–83.

Latour, Bruno. *We Have Never Been Modern.* Translated by Catherine Porter. Cambridge, Mass.: Harvard University Press, 1993.

Leavitt, Judith. *Typhoid Mary: Captive to the Public's Health.* Boston: Beacon, 1996.

Lederberg, Joshua. "Infectious Disease—A Threat to Global Health and Security." *Journal of the American Medical Association* 276, no. 5 (August 7, 1996): 417–19.

———. "Viruses and Humankind: Intracellular Symbiosis and Evolutionary Competition." In *Emerging Viruses*, edited by Stephen S. Morse, 3–9. New York: Oxford University Press, 1993.

Lederberg, Joshua, Robert E. Shope, and Stanley C. Oaks, Jr. *Emerging Infections: Microbial Threats to Health in the United States.* Washington, D.C.: National Academy Press, 1992.

Lewis, Steven. *The Race against Time.* Concord, Ont.: House of Anansi Press, 2006.

Lippens, Ronnie. "Viral Contagion and Anti-terrorism: Notes on Medical Emergency, Legality and Diplomacy." *International Journal for the Semiotics of Law* 17, no. 2 (June 2004): 125–39.

Long, A. A., and D. N. Sedley. *The Hellenistic Philosophers.* Vol. 1, *Translations of the Principal Sources, with Philosophical Commentary.* Cambridge: Cambridge University Press, 1987.

Longmuir, Anne. "Performing the Body in Don DeLillo's *The Body Artist.*" *Modern Fiction Studies* 53, no. 3 (Fall 2007): 529–33.

Los Angeles Times. "TB Terror." June 10, 2007.

Maberry, Jonathan. *Patient Zero.* New York: St. Martin's Press, 2009.

Mackenzie, Debora. "Bird Flu Outbreak Started a Year Ago." *New Scientist* 181, no. 2432 (January 31, 2004): 10–11.

Marsden, Paul. "Memetics and Social Contagion: Two Sides of the Same Coin?" *Journal of Memetics—Evolutionary Models of Information Transmission* 2, no. 2 (1998): 171–85.

Massumi, Brian. "Fear (the Spectrum Said)." *Positions* 12, no. 1 (2005): 31–48.

———. *Parables for the Virtual.* Durham, N.C.: Duke University Press, 2002.

Matheson, Richard. *I Am Legend.* 1954; New York: ORB, 1995.

Mayer, Ruth. "Virus Discourse: The Rhetoric of Threat and Terrorism in the Biothriller." *Cultural Critique* 66 (2007): 1–20.

McClintock, Anne. *Imperial Leather: Race, Gender and Sexuality in the Colonial Conquest.* London: Routledge, 1995.

McDermott, Rose, James H. Fowler, and Nicholas A. Christakis. "Breaking Up Is Hard to Do, Unless Everyone Else Is Doing It Too: Social Network Effects on Divorce in a Longitudinal Sample Followed for 32 Years." October 18, 2009, SSRN. http://ssrn.com/abstract=1490708.

McNeil, Donald G., Jr. "In Daylong Drill, an Agency Tries to Prepare for a Real Outbreak of Avian Flu." *New York Times,* February 1, 2007.

McNeill, William. *Plagues and Peoples.* Garden City, N.J.: Anchor Press, 1976.

Mendelsohn, Andrew. "'Typhoid Mary' Strikes Again: The Social and the Scientific in the Making of Public Health." *Isis* 86, no. 2 (June 1995): 268–77.

Messud, Claire. *The Emperor's Children.* New York: Alfred A. Knopf, 2006.

Milburn, Colin. "Monsters in Eden: Darwin and Derrida." *Modern Language Notes* 118, no. 3 (April 2003): 603–21.

Morley, Catherine. "Don DeLillo's Transatlantic Dialogue with Sergei Eisenstein." *Journal of American Studies* 40, no. 1 (2006): 17–34.

Morse, Stephen S. "Epidemiologic Surveillance for Investigating Chemical or Biological Warfare and for Improving Human Health." *Politics and the Life Sciences* 11, no. 1 (February 1992): 28–29.

———. "The Globalization of Infectious Diseases." Talk delivered at the Whitman College Global Studies Symposium on Contagion, February 27, 2009, Walla Walla, Washington.

————, ed. *Emerging Viruses*. New York: Oxford University Press, 1993.

Mouffe, Chantal. "Hegemony and Ideology in Gramsci." In *Gramsci and Marxist Theory*, 168–204. London: Routledge and Kegan Paul, 1979.

Nancy, Jean-Luc. *Corpus*. Paris: Métailié, 2000.

————. *The Inoperative Community*. Edited by Peter Conor. Translated by Peter Conor, Lisa Garbus, Michael Holland, and Simona Sawhney. Foreword by Christopher Fynsk. Minneapolis: University of Minnesota Press, 1991.

————. *The Sense of the World*. Translated and with a foreword by Jeffrey S. Librett. Minneapolis: University of Minnesota Press, 1997.

National Commission on Terrorist Attacks. *The 9/11 Commission Report: Final Report of the National Commission on Terrorist Attacks upon the United States*. New York: W. W. Norton, 2004.

Nel, Philip. *The Avant-Garde and American Postmodernity: Small Incisive Shots*. Jackson: University of Mississippi Press, 2002.

Neocleous, Mark. "The Problem with Normality: Taking Exception to 'Permanent Emergency.'" *Alternatives: Global, Local, Political* 31, no. 2 (2006): 191–213.

Nguyen, Vinh-Kim. "Antiretroviral Globalism, Biopolitics, and Therapeutic Citizenship." In *Global Assemblages, Technology, Politics and Ethics as Anthropological Problems*, edited by Aihwa Ong and Stephen J. Collier, 124–44. London: Blackwell, 2005.

Nietzsche, Friedrich. *Thus Spoke Zarathustra: A Book for Everyone and No One*. Translated and with an introduction by R. J. Hollingdale. New York: Penguin, 1969.

Oldstone, Michael. *Viruses, Plagues, and History*. New York: Oxford University Press, 1998.

Osterholm, Michael. "Preparing for the Next Pandemic." *Foreign Affairs*, July–August 2005.

Outbreak. Directed by Wolfgang Petersen. DVD. Burbank, Calif.: Warner Brothers, 1995.

Pálsson, Gísli, and Paul Rabinow. "The Iceland Controversy: Reflections on the Transnational Market of Civic Virtue" In *Global Assemblages, Technology, Politics and Ethics as Anthropological Problems*, edited by Aihwa Ong and Stephen J. Collier, 91–103. London: Blackwell, 2005.

Press, Bill. "Press: The Sad Legacy of Jerry Falwell." *Millford Daily News*, May 18, 2007.

Preston, Richard. *The Cobra Event*. New York: Ballantine, 1998.

————. *The Hot Zone*. New York: Doubleday, 1994.

Rabinow, Paul. "Midst Anthropology's Problems." In *Global Assemblages: Technology, Politics and Ethics as Anthropological Problems*, edited by Aihwa Ong and Stephen J. Collier, 40–53. London: Blackwell, 2005.

Rancière, Jacques. *The Politics of Aesthetics: The Distribution of the Sensible.* New York: Continuum, 2004.

Roett, Riordan, and Russell Crandall. "The Global Economic Crisis, Contagion, and Institutions: New Realities in Latin America and Asia." *International Political Science Review* 20, no. 3 (1999): 271–83.

Rose, Nikolas. *The Politics of Life Itself: Biomedicine, Power and Subjectivity in the Twenty-first Century.* Princeton, N.J.: Princeton University Press, 2007.

Rose, Nikolas, and Carlos Novas. "Biological Citizenship." In *Global Assemblages: Technology, Politics and Ethics as Anthropological Problems,* edited by Aihwa Ong and Stephen J. Collier, 439–63. London: Blackwell, 2005.

Rosen, George. *A History of Public Health.* Baltimore, Md.: Johns Hopkins University Press, 1993.

Rosenberg, Charles. "Pathologies of Progress: The Idea of Civilization as Risk." *Bulletin of the History of Medicine* 72, no. 4 (1998): 714–30.

Rothberg, Michael. "A Failure of the Imagination: Diagnosing the Post-9/11 Novel: A Response to Richard Gray." *American Literary History* 21, no. 1 (2009): 152–58.

Ryan, Frank. *Virus X: Tracking the New Killer Plagues — Out of the Present and into the Future.* Boston: Little, Brown, 1997.

Sampson, Tony D. "Contagion Theory beyond the Microbe (and perhaps beyond networks too)." http://www.networkpolitics.org/request-for-comments/dr-thackers-position-paper.

Scheper-Hughes, Nancy. "The Last Commodity: Post-human Ethics and the Global Traffic in 'Fresh' Organs." In *Global Assemblages, Technology, Politics and Ethics as Anthropological Problems,* edited by Aihwa Ong and Stephen J. Collier, 145–67. London: Blackwell, 2005.

Schmitt, Carl. *The Concept of the Political.* Chicago: University of Chicago Press, 1996.

———. *Political Theology.* Cambridge, Mass.: MIT Press, 1985.

Schwartz, John. "Tangle of Conflicting Accounts in TB Patient's Odyssey." *New York Times,* June 2, 2007.

Schwartz, Nelson. "Rumsfeld's Growing Stake in Tamiflu." CNNMoney.com, October 31, 2005. http://money.cnn.com/2005/10/31/news/newsmakers/fortune_rumsfeld/.

Sciolino, Elaine. "Europe Struggling to Train New Breed of Muslim Clerics." *New York Times,* October 18, 2004.

Shah, Nayan. *Contagious Divides: Epidemics and Race in San Francisco's Chinatown.* Berkeley: University of California Press, 2001.

Smart, Barry. *Facing Modernity: Ambivalence, Reflexivity, and Modernity.* London: Sage, 1999.

Smith, Daniel W. Introduction to *Francis Bacon: The Logic of Sensation,* by Gilles Deleuze. Minneapolis: University of Minnesota Press, 2002.

Soper, George A. "The Curious Career of Typhoid Mary." *Bulletin of the New York Academy of Medicine* 15, no. 6 (June 1939): 698–717.

Spanneut, Michel. *Permanence du stoïcisme: De Zénon à Malraux.* Gembloux, Belgium: Duculot, 1973.

Specter, Michael. "Nature's Bioterrorist: Is There Any Way to Prevent a Deadly Avian-Flu Pandemic?" *New Yorker,* February 28, 2005.

Spruyt, Hendrik. *The Sovereign State and Its Competitors.* Princeton, N.J.: Princeton University Press, 1994.

Star Trek: Nemesis. Directed by Stuart Baird. DVD. Hollywood, Calif.: Paramount Home Entertainment, 2002.

Stein, Rob. "Millions of H1N1 Vaccine Doses May Have to Be Discarded." *Washington Post,* April 1, 2010.

Tavernise, Sabrina. "Marines See Signs Iraq Rebels Are Battling Foreign Fighters." *New York Times,* June 21, 2005.

Thacker, Eugene. *Biomedia.* Minneapolis: University of Minnesota Press, 2004.

———. "On the Horror of Living Networks." http://www.networkpolitics.org/request-for-comments/dr-thackers-position-paper.

———. "Cryptobiologies." In Organicities, online node, *Artnodes,* no. 6, UOC. http://www.uoc.edu/ortnodes/6/dt/eng/thacker.pdf. (ISSN 1695–5951).

Tomes, Nancy. *The Gospel of Germs: Men, Women, and the Microbe in American Life.* Cambridge, Mass.: Harvard University Press, 1998.

"'Typhoid Mary' Has Reappeared." *New York Times,* sec. 5, April 4, 1915.

United Nations Economic and Social Council. "Crisis of Human Environment." In *Report of the Secretary-General on Problems of the Human Environment,* 47th session, agenda item 10, May 26, 1969.

Versluys, Kristiaan. *Out of the Blue: September 11 and the Novel.* New York: Columbia University Press, 2009.

Virilio, Paul. *Art and Fear.* London: Continuum, 2004.

Wald, Priscilla. *Contagious: Cultures, Carriers, and the Outbreak Narrative.* Durham, N.C.: Duke University Press, 2008.

Walsh, Bryan. "Indonesia's Bird Flu Showdown." *Time,* May 10, 2007.

Warner, Marina. *Phantasmagoria: Spirit Visions, Metaphors, and Media into the Twenty-first Century.* Oxford: Oxford University Press, 2006.

Weir, Lorna, and Eric Mykhalovskiy. "The Geopolitics of Global Public Health Surveillance in the 21st Century." In *Medicine at the Border: Disease, Globalization, and Security, 1850 to the Present,* edited by Alison Bashford, 240–63. New York: Palgrave Macmillan, 2006.

Whalen, Jeanne, and David Guthier-Villars. "European Governments Cancel Vaccine Orders." *Wall Street Journal,* January 13, 2010.

Whitehall, Geoffrey. "Infected Life and Viral Politics: Agamben and the Avian Flu." Paper presented at the Canada Research Chair in Sustainability and Culture Conference, Toronto, 2007.

————. "Viral Politics: Avian Flu, Difference and Contagion." Paper presented at the 48th Annual Convention of the International Studies Association, Chicago, 2007.

"WHO Warns of Dire Flu Pandemic." CNN. http://www.cnn.com/2004/Health/11/25/birdflu.warning/.

Wiktorowicz, Quintan. "The New Global Threat: Transnational Salafis and Jihad." *Middle East Policy* 8, no. 4 (December 2001): 18–38.

Wills, Christopher. *Yellow Fever, Black Goddess: The Coevolution of People and Plagues.* Reading, Mass.: Addison-Wesley, 1996.

Wilson, Rob, and Arlif Dirlik. *Asia/Pacific as Space of Cultural Production.* Durham, N.C.: Duke University Press, 1995.

Wolfe, Cary. *Animal Rites.* Chicago: Chicago University Press, 2003.

————, ed. *Zoontologies: The Question of the Animal.* Minneapolis: University of Minnesota Press, 2003.

————. "Ten Concerns If Avian Influenza Becomes a Pandemic." http://www.who.int/csr/disease/influenza/pandemic10things/en/.

————. *The World Health Report 2007: A Safer Future; Global Public Health Security in the 21st Century.* Geneva: WTO, 2007.

Wright, Susan. "Terrorists and Biological Weapons." *Politics and the Life Sciences* 25, no. 1 (2006): 57–115.

Wulf, Herbert, and Tobias Debiel. "Conflict Early Warning and Response Mechanisms: Tools for Enhancing the Effectiveness of Regional Organisations? A Comparative Study of the AU, ECOWAS, IGAD, ASEAN/ARF and PIF." Working Paper no. 49. Crisis States Research Centre, London School of Economics Development Studies Institute, May 2009.

Yoo, John. "War, Responsibility, and the Age of Terrorism." *Stanford Law Review* 57, no. 3 (2004): 793–816.

Zeller, Eduard. *The Stoics, Epicureans, and Sceptics.* Translated by Oswald J. Reichel. Rev. ed. New York: Russell & Russell, 1962.

Zinsser, Hans. *Rats, Lice and History.* Boston: Little, Brown and Co., 1935.

Žižek, Slavoj. "20 Years of Collapse." *New York Times*, November 9, 2009. http://www.nytimes.com/2009/11/09/opinion/09zizek.html.

NOTES ON CONTRIBUTORS

Alberto S. Galindo is Assistant Professor of Spanish. He earned his Ph.D. in Spanish and Portuguese Languages and Cultures from Princeton University. His teaching and research interests include post-9/11 literature and culture, Latina/Latino studies, Hispanic Caribbean literatures, race and ethnic studies, English-Spanish translation, and HIV/AIDS and health care.

Andrew Lakoff is Associate Professor of Anthropology, Communications, and Sociology at the University of Southern California. His main areas of interest include science and technology studies, biomedicine, social theory, and globalization processes. Lakoff's first book, *Pharmaceutical Reason: Knowledge and Value in Global Psychiatry* (2005), examines the role of the global circulation of pharmaceuticals in the spread of biological models of human behavior. He also coedited *Global Pharmaceuticals: Ethics, Markets, Practice* (2006) and has published articles on visual technology and the behavioral sciences, the history of attention deficit disorder, and the placebo effect. His current research concerns global health and biosecurity, and his most recent publication is *Biosecurity Interventions: Global Health and Security in Question* (2008), coedited with Stephen J. Collier.

Bruce Magnusson is Associate Professor of Politics and Director of Global Studies at Whitman College. His teaching and research interests are in international, transnational, and comparative politics, with a particular focus on Africa. His work has been published in *Comparative Politics* and *Comparative Studies in Society and History* as well as in multiple volumes on comparative and African politics. Magnusson's current research addresses questions at the intersections of ethnicity, security, violence, and justice in Africa, the politics of ethnic and religious ascription in population censuses in colonial and postcolonial Africa, and elections and censuses as vectors of violence.

Christian Moraru is Professor of English at University of North Carolina, Greensboro. He specializes in critical theory and post–World War II American literature as well as comparative literature with particular emphasis on the history of ideas, narrative, postmodernism in cross-cultural perspective, new material studies, and the relations between globalism, community, and culture. His latest books include *Rewriting: Postmodern Narrative and Cultural Critique in the Age of Cloning* (2001), *Memorious Discourse: Reprise and Representation in Postmodernism* (2005), *Cosmodernism: American Narrative, Late Globalization, and the New Cultural Imaginary* (2010), and the collection *Postcommunism, Postmodernism, and the Global Imagination* (2009).

Paul B. Stares is the General John W. Vessey Senior Fellow for Conflict Prevention and Director of the Center for Preventive Action at the Council on Foreign Relations, where he oversees the Center's series of Contingency Planning Memoranda and Council Special Reports on potential sources of instability and conflict.

Priscilla Wald is Professor of English and Women's Studies at Duke University. She teaches and works on U.S. literature and culture, particularly literature of the late-eighteenth to mid-twentieth centuries. Her current work focuses on the intersections of law, literature, science, and medicine. Wald's book *Contagious: Cultures, Carriers, and the Outbreak Narrative* (2008) considers the conjunction of medicine and myth in the idea of contagion and the evolution of the stories we tell about the global health problem of emerging infections. She is currently working on a book entitled *Human Being After Genocide*, which explores the challenges to the question of the human in science and social thought in the period following World War II, the emergence of science fiction as a recognizable genre, and the rewriting of human history through genetics. Wald is the author of *Constituting Americans: Cultural Anxiety and Narrative Form* (1995), the editor of the journal *American Literature*, and co-editor of a book series on nineteenth-century American literature. She is a member of Duke's Institute for Genome

Sciences and Policy, an affiliate of Duke's Trent Center for Medical Ethics and Humanities, and serves on the Advisory Board of the Centre for the Humanities and Medicine of the University of Hong Kong.

Geoffrey Whitehall is Associate Professor of Political Science at Acadia University, Nova Scotia. His general research interests include international political theory, contemporary political thought, and discourses of culture and technology. His latest publications include "Preemptive Sovereignty and Avian Pandemics," in Theory & Event (2010); "Opening Global Politics: A New Introduction" (cowritten with Rachel Brickner), in International Studies Perspective (2009); "Politics after the Event: Exceeding Asia/Pacific," in Borderlands (2007); and "Musical Modulations of Political Thought: amplifying difference beyond the grammar of sovereignty," in Theory & Event (2006). He is currently working on his book Global Triage: From Sovereignty to Pre-emptive Governance.

Mona Yacoubian joined the Stimson Center in 2011, where she serves as Senior Advisor, Middle East and as Project Director, Pathways to Progress (Middle East/Southwest Asia). She previously served as a Special Advisor and Senior Program Officer on the Middle East at the US Institute of Peace, where her work focused on Lebanon and Syria as well as on broader issues related to democratization in the Arab world.

Zahi Zalloua is Associate Professor of French and General Studies at Whitman College and editor of *The Comparatist*. He is the author of *Montaigne and the Ethics of Skepticism* (2005) and editor of *Montaigne after Theory/Theory after Montaigne* (2009). He has also edited issues of *L'Esprit Créateur* (2006) and *SubStance* (2009) and coedited, with Nicole Simek, a special issue of *Dalhousie French Studies* on representations of trauma in French and Francophone literature (2007). Zalloua's other publications address globalization, literary theory, interdisciplinary approaches to philosophy and literature, experimental fiction, and gender studies. He is currently writing a study on unruly fictions in modern French texts.

INDEX

A

ABC drama, 87, 90, 109

Abraham, Jill, 169n5

Adbusters magazine, 97n82

aesthetic representations, in preemptive emergency creation, 72–79

affective-oriented governance, in preemptive emergency creation, 10, 18–19, 75–79, 86–91

Agamben, Giorgio, 71, 80, 85, 89

Agence France-Presse, 48

agent component, epidemic model, 30–32. *See also* Islamist militancy, counter-epidemic model

Ahmed, Fatema, 169n5

AIDS, 22n11, 55, 57, 63, 90–91, 110

Alma-Ata statement, Chan's, 118, 122n40

al Qaeda, 27, 28

Americanism theme, 13–14, 22n15, 154–55, 164–65, 171n22

American Political Science Association, 95n43

"American Prose Writing at a Time of Crisis" (Gray), 152

Amis, Martin, 152, 172nn48–49

Anderson, Benedict, 166

Anderson, Warwick, 68n29

Angelus Novus (Klee), 87–88

APEC Health Task Force, 78, 82–83, 86

Arabs, fictional criticisms, 163, 172n50

art reproduction, in DeLillo's novels, 132–35, 138–44

Asian Pacific Economic Cooperation (APEC), 78, 82–83, 86

195

69, 171n29, n31, 172nn33–34, n52
London, 28, 43n9
Los Angeles Times, 61
love arguments, 23n27
Low, Donald, 76
Ludovic, in *The Emperor's Children*, 154, 171n16

M

Maberry, Jonathan, 12, 99–100, 111
Madrid attacks, 28
Magnusson, Bruce: biographical highlights, 190; chapter by, 3–23
malaria, 52, 90
Mallon, Mary, 103–4
mapping representations, influenza threat, 77–78
Mariella, in *The Body Artist*, 143
Marina Thwaite, in *The Emperor's Children*, 154
Masri, Abu Hamza Al-, 43n9
Massumi, Brian, 75, 89–90
Matheson, Richard, 107, 112–13, 117
McNeil, Donald, Jr., 87
media, in *The Believers*, 159, 172n34
medicalized nativism, 103
Messud, Claire. *See The Emperor's Children* (Messud)
Miami, in *The Emperor's Children*, 155, 171n22
microbe monsters. *See* biohorror narratives
Mike, in *The Believers*, 163
Milburn, Colin, 113–14
Mohammed Hassani, in *The Believers*, 158–66, 171n29
The Monitor, in *The Emperor's Children*, 154–55
monsters. *See* biohorror narratives
Moraru, Christian: biographical high-

lights, 190; chapter by, 123–48; comments on, 16–17, 19–20
Morse, Stephen S., 5–6, 54, 68n36
Mouffe, Chantal, 170n8
Murray Thwaite, in *The Emperor's Children* (Messud), 149–50, 151, 153–57, 156
myth. *See* bourgeois liberalism, in post-9/11 novels

N

The Names (DeLillo), 131
Nancy, Jean-Luc, 125–27, 130, 145
narrative construction. *See* biohorror narratives; bourgeois liberalism, in post-9/11 novels; culture, haptical theory of; preemptive emergency state, influenza threat
nationalist insurgent groups, as Islamist militancy constituency, 27
nativism, 20n1, 103, 113
nature's revenge perspective, 10–11, 22n11
necrophiliac pornography, 154, 171n16
Negri, Antonio, 12, 23n27
Netherland (O'Neill), 153
network theory, 21n3
Neville, Richard, in *I Am Legend*, 112–13, 117
New Scientist, 91
New York City, crime control approach, 42n6
New York Times, 61, 87
Nick, in *Underworld*, 134, 136–37
Nietzsche, 125
9/11 attacks, 14, 25. *See also* Islamist militancy, counter-epidemic model; terrorism

timing question, in *The Emperor's Children*, 157

tipping points, 30, 42n6

transnational jihadist groups, in counter-epidemic model, 27, 31–32, 34, 35–36

Tubb, Frederick, in *The Emperor's Children*, 154

tuberculosis, 61–62, 69n51, 90

Tuttle, in *The Body Artist*, 140–43

Typhoid Mary, 103–4

U

Underworld (DeLillo), 16, 131, 133–37

Unterwelt (Eisentein), 135, 138

V

vaccine programs: counterterrorism comparison, 33–34, 36–37; H1N1 virus threat, 64–65; in H5N1 sovereignty conflict, 9, 47–48, 49–50; public health system history, 52, 67n18; triage approach, 84–85

vampire narratives, 100, 112–13, 117

vectors component, epidemic model, 30–32. *See also* Islamist militancy, counter-epidemic model

Versluys, Kristiaan, 150

viral contagion, global perspective origins, 5–7. *See also specific topics, e.g.,* biohorror narratives; culture, haptical theory of; global health security, preparedness framework

Virilio, Paul, 87

Virus X: Tracking the New Killer Plagues (Ryan), 10–11

W

Wald, Priscilla: biographical high-

lights, 190–91; chapter by, 99–122; comments on, 11–12, 19, 170n7

Warner, Marina, 113

Washington Post, 45–46, 64

Whitehall, Geoffrey: biographical highlights, 191; chapter by, 71–98; comments on, 8, 9–10, 15, 18–19

WHO. *See* World Health Organization (WHO)

wire transfers, as viral revolution, 128

Wodarg, Wolfgang, 65

World Bank, 53

World Health Organization (WHO): Alma-Ata Declaration, 118, 122n40; disease risk report, 53–55, 67n25; H1N1 virus threat, 63–64, 65; H5N1 sovereignty conflict, 46–48; international health efforts, 52–53; pandemic representations, 77, 79; regulatory framework, 48–50, 57–59

World Wide Web, in *Underworld*, 135–36

Wright, Susan, 68n33, 109–10

X

XDR-TB case, 61–62

Y

Yacoubian, Mona: biographical highlights, 191; chapter by, 25–43; comments on, 5, 7, 18

Yoo, John, 14

Z

Zalloua, Zahi: biographical highlights, 191; chapter by, 3–23

Zero, in *The Blood Artists*, 107–8

Žižek, Slavoj, 127

CPSIA information can be obtained at www.ICGtesting.com
Printed in the USA
BVOW040403210512

290635BV00001B/11/P